Diversity, Equity, and Inclusion in Veterinary Medicine, Part I

Editor

CHRISTINA V. TRAN

VETERINARY CLINICS
OF NORTH AMERICA:
SMALL ANIMAL PRACTICE

www.vetsmall.theclinics.com

September 2024 • Volume 54 • Number 5

ELSEVIER
1600 John F. Kennedy Boulevard • Suite 1800 • Philadelphia, Pennsylvania, 19103-2899
http://www.vetsmall.theclinics.com

VETERINARY CLINICS OF NORTH AMERICA: SMALL ANIMAL PRACTICE Volume 54, Number 5 September 2024 ISSN 0195-5616, ISBN-13: 978-0-443-29718-2

Editor: Stacy Eastman
Developmental Editor: Varun Gopal

Veterinary Clinics of North America: Small Animal Practice (ISSN 0195-5616) is published bimonthly by Elsevier Inc., 360 Park Avenue South, New York, NY 10010-1710. Months of issue are January, March, May, July, September, and November. Business and Editorial Offices: 1600 John F. Kennedy Blvd., Ste. 1800, Philadelphia, PA 19103-2899. Customer Service Office: 3251 Riverport Lane, Maryland Heights, MO 63043. Periodicals postage paid at New York, NY and additional mailing offices. Subscription prices are $391.00 per year (domestic individuals), $100.00 per year (domestic students/residents), $503.00 per year (Canadian individuals), $544.00 per year (international individuals), $100.00 per year (Canadian students/residents), and $220.00 per year (international students/residents). For institutional access pricing please contact Customer Service via the contact information below. To receive student/resident rate, orders must be accompained by name of affiliated institution, date of term, and the *signature* of program/residency coordinator on institution letterhead. Orders will be billed at individual rate until proof of status is received. Foreign air speed delivery is included in all *Clinics* subscription prices. All prices are subject to change without notice. Orders, claims, and journal inquiries: Please visit our Support Hub page https://service.elsevier.com for assistance.

Reprints. For copies of 100 or more of articles in this publication, please contact the Commercial Reprints Department, Elsevier Inc., 360 Park Avenue South, New York, NY 10010-1710. Tel.: 212-633-3874; Fax: 212-633-3820; E-mail: reprints@elsevier.com.

Veterinary Clinics of North America: Small Animal Practice is also published in Japanese by Inter Zoo Publishing Co., Ltd., Aoyama Crystal-Bldg 5F, 3-5-12 Kitaaoyama, Minato-ku, Tokyo 107-0061, Japan.

Veterinary Clinics of North America: Small Animal Practice is covered in *Current Contents/Agriculture, Biology and Environmental Sciences, Science Citation Index, ASCA, MEDLINE/PubMed (Index Medicus), Excerpta Medica, and BIOSIS.*

Contributors

EDITOR

CHRISTINA V. TRAN, DVM
Founding Dean and Clinical Professor, School of Veterinary Medicine, Hanover College, Hanover, Indiana, USA; Past President and Founding Board Member, Multicultural Veterinary Medical Association, Silverdale, Washington, USA

AUTHORS

CORLICE ATKINS, JD
Executive Director, Vet for a Day, Bonaire, Georgia, USA

KATHERINE FOGELBERG, DVM, PhD
Regional Doctor Mentor, Thrive Pet Healthcare, Austin, Texas, USA

VERNARD HODGES, DVM
Bonaire, Georgia, USA; Owner, Critter Fixer Veterinary Hospital, Warner Robins, Georgia, USA

SOHAILA JAFARIAN, DVM, MPH
Board Member for the Multicultural Veterinary Medical Association, Relief Veterinarian for Jafarian Relief Services, LLC, Albuquerque, New Mexico, USA

AMBER LABELLE, DVM, MS
Diplomate of the American College of Veterinary Ophthalmologists; Practice Owner and Veterinary Ophthalmologist, Bright Light Veterinary Eye Care, Ottawa, Ontario, Canada

MELODY MARTÍNEZ, CVT
President of the Multicultural Veterinary Medical Association (MCVMA), Founder and Principal, Acorde Consulting; Medical Committee Member, Portland Animal Welfare Team

CHARLES D. McMILLAN, DVM
Medical Director and Owner, GoodVets West Buckhead, Atlanta, Georgia, USA

STEPHEN NIÑO CITAL, RVT, SRA, RLAT, CVPP, VTS-LAM (Research Anesthesia)
Lab Manager, Department of Neurobiology, Stanford University, Stanford, California, USA; Chief Veterinary Nursing Officer, Remedy Veterinary Specialists, San Francisco, California, USA

GEORGE ROBINSON, DVM, MSPH
Founder and Former CEO, Heartland Veterinary Partners, LLC, Miromar Lakes, Florida, USA

JEAN-YIN TAN, DVM, MBA
Diplomate of the American College of Veterinary Internal Medicine; Associate Professor (Teaching), University of Calgary Faculty of Veterinary Medicine, Calgary, Alberta, Canada

SUSAN M. WILLIAMS, DVM, PhD
American College of Poultry Veterinarians, Professor and Interim Assistant Dean for Diversity, Equity and Inclusion, Department of Population Health, Poultry Diagnostic and Research Center, College of Veterinary Medicine, University of Georgia, Athens, Georgia, USA

Contents

VETERINARY CLINICS OF NORTH AMERICA: SMALL ANIMAL PRACTICE

FORTHCOMING ISSUES

November 2024
Diversity, Equity, and Inclusion in Veterinary Medicine, Part II
Christina V. Tran, *Editor*

January 2025
Update on Diagnosis and Treatment of Brain Tumors in Dogs and Cats
Helena Rylander, *Editor*

March 2025
Small Animal Dermatology
Bailey Brame and Peter Canning, *Editors*

RECENT ISSUES

July 2024
Small Animal Endoscopy
Boel A. Fransson, *Editor*

May 2024
Small Animal Oncology
Craig A. Clifford and Philip J. Bergman, *Editors*

March 2024
Practice Management
Peter Weinstein, *Editor*

Preface

A Work in Progress: Diversity, Equity, and Inclusion Challenges and Opportunities Within Veterinary Medicine

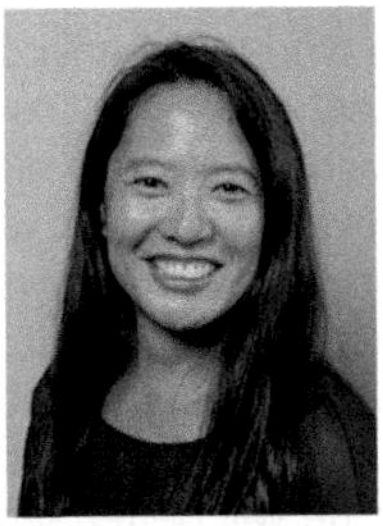

Christina V. Tran, DVM
Editor

In recent years, the veterinary profession has faced increasing calls for greater diversity, equity, and inclusion (DEI). As our society evolves and becomes more aware of systemic inequalities, it is imperative that all professional fields, including veterinary medicine, reflect these changes. For the first time, *Veterinary Clinics of North America: Small Animal Practice* has published two issues exploring DEI within the context of veterinary medicine, a field that has historically lagged behind others in addressing these critical issues.

Veterinary medicine is a diverse field that includes not only veterinarians but also veterinary technicians, assistants, researchers, educators, and administrators. Each of these roles plays a crucial part in the overall health and well-being of animals and the advancement of veterinary science. However, despite the diversity of roles, the demographic makeup of the veterinary profession has not kept pace with the changing demographics of society at large. This lack of diversity has profound implications for the quality of care provided, the accessibility of veterinary services, and the well-being of those working within the profession.

The articles in this issue aim to provide a broad examination of some of the DEI challenges and opportunities within veterinary medicine. We begin by exploring the current state of diversity within the profession, drawing on statistical data as well as lived experience, from both veterinarians and veterinary technicians. This foundation is essential for understanding where we are and what progress still needs to be made. It is clear that more research, including qualitative research, is needed to fully realize what changes are needed to address DEI in veterinary medicine. Subsequent articles delve

Vet Clin Small Anim 54 (2024) ix–x
https://doi.org/10.1016/j.cvsm.2024.06.010

into the barriers that prevent greater diversity, including systemic issues within educational institutions, professional organizations, and workplaces.

One critical area of focus is the educational pipeline. Well before the application process, prospective veterinary students are influenced by their early experiences (or lack thereof) with pet ownership and veterinary role models. Veterinary schools and veterinary technology programs are the entry points into the profession, and the experiences of students in these environments can significantly impact their career trajectories. Several issue articles consider aspects of the pipeline, including community outreach efforts, access to veterinary role models and mentors, the support systems in place for students from underrepresented backgrounds, and the challenges these students face during their education. We also highlight successful initiatives and programs that have made strides in promoting DEI within veterinary medicine.

Another important aspect of DEI in veterinary medicine is the workplace environment. Several issue articles discuss the policies and practices that can either foster or hinder a diverse and inclusive workplace culture. Topics such as implicit bias, practice ownership, and leadership diversity are addressed, providing readers with practical strategies for creating more equitable and inclusive work environments.

As guest editor and contributors, our goal is to inspire and equip current and future veterinary professionals with the knowledge and tools they need to foster a more diverse, equitable, and inclusive profession. By embracing DEI and committing to a sustained effort to address systemic injustices, veterinary medicine will better serve both the animal and the human communities it is dedicated to. This issue is a call to action, encouraging everyone in the veterinary field to educate themselves and actively work toward making DEI a central tenet of their professional practice.

We hope that this collection of articles will not only inform but also motivate readers to take meaningful steps toward creating a veterinary profession that is truly reflective of the diverse society it serves. Thank you for joining us on this important journey toward equity and inclusion in veterinary medicine.

DISCLOSURES

The author has no conflicts of interest to disclose.

Christina V. Tran, DVM
School of Veterinary Medicine
Hanover College
517 Ball Drive
Hanover, IN, USA

Multicultural Veterinary Medical Association
Silverdale, Washington, USA

E-mail address:
tran@hanover.edu

Understanding the Why

The Need for Diversity, Equity, and Inclusion in Veterinary Medicine

Melody Martínez, CVT[a,b,c,*]

KEYWORDS

• Diversity • Equity • Inclusion • Belonging • Race • Discrimination • Bias • Ethnicity

KEY POINTS

- Veterinary medicine is one of the most white-dominated professions in the United States, highlighting a significant lack of racial diversity.
- Historical injustices, such as colonial violence, enslavement, and exclusionary laws, have created systemic barriers that continue to affect marginalized communities, including within the veterinary profession.
- The high cost of education and significant debt burden relative to starting salaries disproportionately affect people of color limiting access to veterinary careers.
- Childhood experiences with animals play a role in motivating individuals to pursue veterinary careers. Lower pet ownership rates among people of color affect career entry.
- Discrimination against veterinary professionals and clients of color lead to higher turnover rates and subpar care for pets, highlighting the need for increased racial diversity.

INTRODUCTION

All professional industries in the United States face challenges with racial diversity, equity, and inclusion. Broadly and plainly speaking, this is a result of a history of colonial settler violence including the genocide of Native Americans, enslavement of Africans, exclusionary laws against people of color, and many other acts of injustice. These historical injustices have created systemic barriers that continue to affect marginalized communities today. While we cannot change the past, it is our duty and responsibility to work toward a better future.

Even within this broader context, why is the veterinary profession so especially White? In fact, veterinary medicine is one of the most White-dominated professions in the country. According to the Bureau of Labor and Statistics, as of 2023, approximately 90% of veterinarians and veterinary technicians and 86% of veterinary assistants in the United

[a] Multicultural Veterinary Medical Association (MCVMA); [b] Acorde Consulting; [c] Portland Animal Welfare Team

* Corresponding author. 2355 State Street, Suite 101, Salem, OR 97301.

E-mail address: MelodyMartinezCVT@gmail.com

Vet Clin Small Anim 54 (2024) 753–765

https://doi.org/10.1016/j.cvsm.2024.06.009 vetsmall.theclinics.com

0195-5616/24/

States are White, a statistic highlighting the severe lack of racial diversity in this field.[1] Most causes are financial in nature and rooted in the racial wealth gap. However, other complex factors are widely understood to contribute to this outcome.

The financial barriers include the high cost of veterinary education and the significant debt burden relative to starting salaries, which disproportionately affect people of color. Additionally, media representations and workplace cultures often do not reflect the racial diversity of the broader population, further discouraging people of color from pursuing careers in veterinary medicine.

Identifying problems is the easy part—working to fix them is the real challenge. This article lays the foundation for the more solution-oriented articles that follow. By understanding the root causes and current challenges, we can develop effective strategies to create a more inclusive and equitable profession for future generations.

LISTENING, BELIEVING, AND ACTING

Meaningfully listening to the experiences of Black, Indigenous, and people of color (BIPOC) in veterinary medicine means actively engaging with their stories, perspectives, and challenges without judgment or dismissal. It requires that we acknowledge the systemic racism, historical barriers, and resulting outcomes that have marginalized BIPOC individuals in the field and validate their lived experiences of discrimination and microaggressions. To do this effectively, we must be willing to learn, unlearn, and challenge our own biases, recognizing that our understanding of the world may be limited by our own cultures, privileges, and experiences.

To truly listen, we must create spaces where BIPOC individuals feel comfortable sharing their stories without fear of retribution, ostracization, or further harm. This means fostering a culture of empathy, compassion, allyship, and solidarity with BIPOC within the veterinary community. It also involves actively amplifying the voices of BIPOC professionals, expanding their leadership opportunities and promoting their presence in leadership spaces, championing their ideas, and materially supporting their initiatives for change.

Additionally, it is imperative that when we seek to understand the experiences of veterinary professionals better—whether to elucidate factors like mental health, financial well-being, workplace satisfaction, and so forth—that we include race, ethnicity, and other social identities in our investigations. By not including race and ethnicity in our investigations of professional experiences, we suggest that racialized experiences do not exist and, by extension, that people of color do not exist in the profession.

Similarly, it is critical to disaggregate the data we obtain by race, ethnicity, skin tone, and socioeconomic factors to better appreciate the unique disparities faced by veterinary professionals of color and those interacting with the profession. When we neglect to analyze data in this way, we essentially obscure or render invisible the experiences of many individuals and whole communities making it impossible to acknowledge disparities and the impacts they create or develop effective solutions to correct them. These oversights also fail to recognize the limitations of sociologic investigations that do not include a complete picture of the veterinary profession's demographics.

This kind of methodology ultimately skews data and their resulting conclusions toward majority experiences and perspectives to the disadvantage of BIPOC and the profession as a whole. Finally, how these data are obtained matters substantially in as much that standard, quantitative research methodology may not effectively capture the nuanced and contextualized stories and experiences of BIPOC individuals and communities, further perpetuating harm and sowing mistrust.[2]

We can only begin to dismantle the systemic inequalities that have historically—and continue to—plague the profession when we listen to, believe, and act on the suggestions made by BIPOC veterinary professionals and clients. The impact of such a simple act of trust is a more inclusive and equitable environment for all, leading to just outcomes and ensuring that every community can benefit from the veterinary profession's contributions to society.

HISTORICAL AND STRUCTURAL BARRIERS

The veterinary profession in the United States has always been very White, and originally this was by design. This homogeneity can also be attributed to several present-day factors, but we cannot ignore the overt exclusionary practices of professional institutions in the past.

The roots of these disparities can be traced back to the early days of veterinary medicine in the United States. The establishment of veterinary schools and professional organizations predominantly catered to White men, excluding women and people of color. After the Civil War, universities were largely segregated, with Black universities "operating with inadequately trained faculty and substandard instructional facilities."[3] These exclusionary practices were not limited to admissions but extended to professional associations and licensing bodies, which often had discriminatory policies that prevented people of color from entering and advancing within the profession.

The introduction of affirmative action helped diversify campuses, but even as other fields attracted more people of color, the veterinary field has stagnated through to the present day. What makes it different from human medicine, where nearly half of doctors are now people of color? We will continue to explore the divergent paths on racial diversity those 2 industries have taken in the modern day.

IMPACT OF CHILDHOOD EXPERIENCES WITH ANIMALS

A deep love and compassion for animals often serve as the primary motivation for individuals pursuing a career in veterinary medicine. The desire to alleviate animal suffering, promote their well-being, and strengthen the human–animal bond resonates strongly with aspiring veterinarians.[4] This passion often stems from early childhood experiences with pets, volunteering at animal shelters, or exposure to veterinary professionals who serve as role models.

If children with exposure to pets are more likely to become veterinarians, it is crucial to examine the demographics of pet ownership in the United States. According to the American Veterinary Medical Association's (AVMA) 2018 *U.S. Pet Ownership and Demographics Sourcebook*, White households in the United States have the highest rate of pet ownership at 68%, followed by Asian households at 57%, Hispanic households at 52%, and Black households at 44%.[5] Compared to a 1983 survey, this represents an increase in pet ownership overall, but the "pet ownership gap" has actually widened. The 1983 study found that 65% of White respondents owned pets compared to 46% of BIPOC respondents.[6]

The methodology for these surveys was different, so we cannot draw direct comparisons, but we can conclude that we have not made significant inroads to diversify pet ownership. Most of today's veterinarians were raised in the 1980s and 1990s when the demographics were likely similar to the 1983 survey. If exposure to animals during childhood is a main driver for joining the industry, progress will likely be slow since the improvement has been minimal. Today's children are tomorrow's veterinarians, and White children continue to have the advantage.

Why exactly are people of color less likely to own pets? While it is possible that cultural norms could play a role—something discussed later in this article—the main cause is likely rooted in economics.

UNDERSTANDING THE RACIAL WEALTH GAP

The racial wealth gap refers to the significant disparity in wealth accumulation among different racial groups in the United States. This gap is not solely a Black/White issue but affects various racial and ethnic groups. While the median White family has nearly 10 times the wealth of the median Black family, other racial and ethnic groups also experience disparities in wealth accumulation compared to their White counterparts.[7] These disparities result from historical and ongoing systemic inequalities that have hindered the economic progress of marginalized communities.

One of the key contributors to the racial wealth gap is the historical legacy of slavery and discriminatory practices that denied people of color access to land ownership, education, and economic opportunities. These historical injustices have had a lasting impact on wealth accumulation, as the disadvantages faced by previous generations continue to affect the economic well-being of their descendants. For example, discriminatory housing policies, like redlining, prevented Black families from purchasing homes in certain neighborhoods, limiting their ability to build wealth through homeownership.[8]

Beyond the legacy of slavery, the Jim Crow era further cemented economic disparities through segregation laws that restricted access to quality education, employment opportunities, and social services. Black Americans and other people of color were systematically excluded from the wealth-building opportunities that White Americans enjoyed, such as access to better schools, stable jobs with benefits, and government programs like the GI Bill, which provided funding for education and home loans primarily to White veterans and their families.

Educational disparities also play a significant role in perpetuating the wealth gap. Schools in predominantly BIPOC neighborhoods often receive less funding, leading to lower quality education and fewer resources. This educational disadvantage can limit access to higher education and high-paying jobs. Additionally, people of color are underrepresented in high-earning industries and overrepresented in low-wage jobs, further exacerbating income inequality.

The cumulative effect of these factors over time has resulted in a significant disparity in wealth between White households and households of color. For instance, a study by the Pew Research Center found that the median wealth of White households was 5.1 times that of Hispanic households and 9.2 times that of Black households.[9] These disparities are not just statistics; they translate into real-world consequences, such as reduced access to quality health care, lower life expectancy, and limited social mobility for future generations.

The racial wealth gap is a deeply entrenched issue rooted in historical and ongoing systemic discrimination. While there are households of color who find themselves in better economic conditions than others and White households who experience economic disenfranchisement, the racial wealth gap is still a driving force in much of our society's outcomes. Addressing this gap is critical for achieving true racial and economic equity, ensuring that all individuals, regardless of race or ethnicity, have the opportunity to thrive and succeed in the United States.

THE MANY PRIVILEGES OF HOME OWNERSHIP

Homeownership has long been considered a cornerstone of wealth accumulation and financial stability in the United States. For people of color, achieving this milestone has been fraught with systemic barriers and discriminatory practices. These barriers are deeply rooted in the country's history and continue to affect the ability of racially marginalized communities to build and sustain wealth.

Even today, despite the 1968 Fair Housing Act, discrimination in the housing market persists.[9] The Fair Housing Act was intended to eliminate discrimination based on race, color, religion, sex, or national origin in the sale, rental, and financing of housing. However, studies have shown that people of color are more likely to be denied mortgages, offered less favorable loan terms, and steered toward less desirable neighborhoods.[10] These discriminatory practices manifest in various ways, including differential treatment by real estate agents, biased appraisals, and inequitable access to credit.

These practices not only limit access to homeownership but also perpetuate the racial wealth gap by hindering the ability of people of color to build equity and pass on wealth to future generations. Homeownership is a primary means through which American families build wealth. The equity gained from owning a home can be used to finance education, start businesses, and provide a financial safety net. When people of color are systematically excluded from homeownership, they are denied these opportunities for wealth accumulation.

As of the fourth quarter of 2023, data reveal that the homeownership rate among non-Hispanic White Americans stood at 73.8%, followed by Asian Americans at 63%, Hispanic Americans at 49.8%, and Black Americans at 45.9%.[11] These statistics highlight a significant racial disparity in homeownership rates, reflecting the ongoing challenges that people of color face in achieving homeownership.

If people of color do not own their homes, they must be renting them. Renting, while providing housing stability for many, does not offer the same wealth-building opportunities as homeownership. Renters are unable to build equity in their homes and are often subject to rising rental costs, which can further limit their ability to save for a down payment on a home.

In many rental properties, a "no pets" policy is a common clause in lease agreements. This restriction often stems from landlords' concerns about potential property damage, noise complaints, and liability issues that pets may cause. Even when rental properties do allow animals, they may have breed or size restrictions that would discourage a renter from getting an animal if they are unable to have the type or breed they want. These policies disproportionately affect people of color, who are already more likely to be renters due to the systemic barriers to homeownership.

As a result, many renters find themselves unable to share their homes with animal companions, even if they are responsible pet owners who would take excellent care of their animals and the property. The inability to own pets can impact the quality of life and emotional well-being of renters, further contributing to the disparities in pet ownership and, by extension, in the veterinary profession.

VETERINARY CARE DESERTS

Poor neighborhoods often receive less capital investment from both government and private businesses, leading to persistent inequalities in resources and opportunities. Historically, policies and practices like redlining, exclusionary zoning, and discriminatory lending have systematically denied Black communities and other people of color access to well-resourced neighborhoods.[12] These practices have led to the geographic concentration of poverty, where essential services like quality schools, health care, grocery stores, and even veterinary offices are lacking. This disinvestment exacerbates economic disparities and hinders upward mobility for residents of these neighborhoods.

The legacy of such discriminatory policies continues to affect present-day investment patterns. Private businesses are less likely to invest in predominantly Black or Latino neighborhoods, further entrenching economic disadvantages. Government investments also tend to favor wealthier, predominantly White neighborhoods, leaving poorer communities with inadequate infrastructure, public services, and economic opportunities. This cycle of disinvestment not only perpetuates poverty but also contributes to broader societal inequities in health, education, and employment outcomes, reinforcing the systemic barriers faced by racially marginalized communities.

In "Access to Veterinary Care: Barriers, Current Practices, and Public Policy," researchers discuss their findings that up to 15% of pet owners reported a lack of transportation as a barrier to veterinary care.[13] If no clinics exist in your neighborhood, traveling to one becomes far more difficult. In urban areas, transportation outside one's neighborhood becomes increasingly burdensome when public transportation policies restrict nonservice animals or animals of a certain size or breed from traveling via public transit, further limiting access to veterinary services.

DOING THE MATH: FINANCIAL CONCERNS ABOUT VETERINARY CAREER PATHS

The veterinary field has had difficulty attracting science, technology, engineering, and mathematics (STEM) students for decades as they opt for careers in human medicine, engineering, and other more lucrative fields.

The cost of veterinary school, while significant, is generally lower than the cost of attending medical school. According to the AVMA, the average tuition for in-state students at veterinary schools in the United States ranges from US$20,000 to US$50,000 per year, with out-of-state tuition being considerably higher.[14] In contrast, the Association of American Medical Colleges reports that the average annual tuition for medical school is approximately US$40,000 to US$60,000 for in-state students and can exceed US$60,000 for out-of-state students.[15] While both veterinary and medical students graduate with substantial debt, the overall cost of veterinary education tends to be lower. However, veterinary students often face a higher debt-to-income ratio compared to medical graduates due to the typically lower starting salaries in the veterinary field.[14]

In addition to tuition costs, both veterinary and medical students incur expenses for books, supplies, living costs, and examination fees. These additional costs can add thousands of dollars annually to the overall expense of their education. Financial aid opportunities, such as scholarships, grants, and loan forgiveness programs, are available for both fields but often do not fully cover the costs. Medical students have better access to these resources due to the larger number of scholarships and loan forgiveness programs available in the health care sector.[14]

According to the AVMA, the average debt for 2022 graduates was US$157,146 for public schools and US$202,468 for private schools, excluding any undergraduate debt.[15] Debt for medical school students is similar, with a median education debt for medical school graduates in 2023 of US$200,000.[1] Despite incurring similar levels of debt for schooling, the average salary of a veterinarian is notably lower than that of a medical doctor. The Bureau of Labor Statistics (BLS) reports a median annual wage of US$100,370 for veterinarians in 2023, compared to US$208,000 for physicians and surgeons in 2021.[16,17] This significant disparity in income exacerbates the debt-to-income ratio for veterinary graduates, making the financial burden more substantial.

Two-year education costs and salaries for nurses and veterinary technicians are similarly disparate. A 2 year program to become a veterinary technician costs at least US$5000. One in-person/on-campus Veterinary Technology program at Portland

Community College in Portland, Oregon, costs an estimated US$13,200 (including general education credits). According to the BLS in 2023, the median annual wage for veterinary technicians and technologists was US$38,460.[18] That is also on par with the wages being offered in Portland.

In comparison, a 2 year nursing degree at the same school in Portland costs US$16,000, while the median annual salary for nurses with 2 year degrees is US$77,000—over double what a veterinary technician earns. This disparity highlights just one of the many reasons the veterinary industry is severely lacking and losing credentialed technicians to medical health care careers. The economic returns of a nursing degree are significantly higher, making it a more attractive option for students and departing veterinary technicians and assistants, especially those from lower income backgrounds.

Research indicates that lower income students are drawn to careers that they perceive as offering stable employment and good wages.[19] Given the financial challenges and lower salary prospects in the veterinary field, it is understandable why fewer BIPOC students or students from economically disadvantaged backgrounds choose this career path.

WELCOME TO THE COUNTRY: RURAL VETERINARY SCHOOLS

The return on investment is not the only thing that sets veterinary programs apart from medical schools: veterinary schools are almost all located in rural areas, while medical schools are predominantly in urban areas.[20] This distinction has significant implications for the racial and ethnic diversity and accessibility of veterinary education.

Establishing veterinary schools in rural areas was initially a practical decision. In the past, veterinary medicine primarily focused on livestock and agricultural animals, which are, of course, found in rural settings.[21] Locating schools in these areas provided easy access to farms and ranches, facilitating hands-on training and research opportunities for students. In modern times, rural communities often face shortages of veterinary professionals,[22] so some argue that keeping schools in these areas can incentivize graduates to stay and serve the local population, addressing workforce needs.

The rural location of veterinary schools can significantly affect admissions. Due to the proximity to agricultural communities and a shortage of agricultural vets, schools may prioritize applicants with agricultural backgrounds or a demonstrated interest in working with livestock.[23] This can inadvertently create a bias against urban applicants who may have less exposure to large animal medicine but possess other valuable skills and interests. Additionally, the limited number of veterinary schools in the country, often clustered in specific regions, can create geographic barriers for applicants, making it difficult for those living far away to attend.[21] A prospective student from a major urban center might find it challenging to relocate to a rural area, both logistically and financially.

The lack of racial and ethnic diversity in rural areas may be reflected in the applicant pool, potentially limiting the number of people of color who apply. According to the Pew Research Center, people in urban areas are 44% White, compared with 68% in suburbs and 79% in rural areas.[20] This demographic trend could mean that rural veterinary schools are likely drawing from a predominantly White potential applicant pool, further perpetuating the lack of diversity in the profession.

The cost of relocating to a rural area and the limited availability of social and cultural amenities can deter some students from applying, particularly those from BIPOC backgrounds who may not feel as comfortable or supported in a rural environment. Urban environments typically offer more cultural amenities, social networks, and opportunities for personal and professional growth, which can be significant factors for students when choosing a school. The rural setting may also lack the support systems and communities that BIPOC students might rely on, making the transition more challenging.

The concentration of veterinary schools in rural areas contrasts sharply with the more evenly distributed or urban-centric locations of medical schools. This difference highlights the varying historical and practical priorities of the 2 fields but also underscores the need for a more strategic approach to veterinary education that considers racial and ethnic diversity and accessibility. Increasing the number of veterinary schools in urban areas and implementing creative, modern solutions to veterinary education such as distance and distributive-hybrid learning and limited licensure options (eg, restricting some veterinary licensing to small animals, reducing the need for large animal education and rural relocation) could help attract a more diverse applicant pool, offering students from all backgrounds the opportunity to pursue veterinary medicine without the additional barriers posed by rural relocation.

A SENSE OF BELONGING

Many students of color report feeling isolated or facing undue pressure as a result of the predominantly White and rural demographic of many veterinary schools.[22] These experiences can significantly impact their academic performance and overall well-being, leading to higher dropout rates and decreased satisfaction with their educational journey.

The lack of diversity among faculty and staff can exacerbate feelings of isolation for students of color. Representation matters, and when students do not see themselves reflected in their educators or mentors, it can be challenging to envision their own success in the field. This lack of diversity can also mean fewer role models and mentors who understand and can address the unique challenges faced by students of color. Mentorship is crucial in guiding students through the complexities of veterinary education and career planning, and without it, students may struggle to navigate these pathways effectively.[24]

A culture of perfectionism, self-sufficiency, and high stress is prevalent in veterinary schools, which can be particularly daunting for students who may already experience marginalization. The intense academic and clinical demands of veterinary programs require a robust support system, and without adequate representation and mentorship, students of color may find it difficult to cope with the pressure. This high-stress environment can lead to burnout, mental health issues, and a feeling of being overwhelmed, further alienating these students.

Microaggressions and subtle forms of discrimination can undermine the confidence and sense of belonging among students of color. These can range from insensitive comments and assumptions about their capabilities or presence to systemic issues such as biased evaluation and grading practices. Such experiences can contribute to a hostile learning environment, making it even harder for these students to succeed.

MEDIA DEPICTIONS OF VETERINARIANS

Veterinarians in popular culture are predominantly depicted as White, which accurately reflects the demographics of the industry but has not helped in efforts to diversify the profession. Media representations play a crucial role in shaping public perceptions and aspirations. When popular media predominantly showcases White veterinarians, it reinforces the notion that veterinary medicine is a field primarily for White individuals, potentially discouraging children of color from considering careers in this field.[25]

For example, Dr Michelle Oakley, the star of the Nat Geo Wild series "Dr. Oakley, Yukon Vet," is a White veterinarian who treats animals in remote areas of Alaska and Canada. Similarly, the NBC sitcom "Animal Practice" featured Dr George Coleman, a White veterinarian played by Justin Kirk, who runs a veterinary clinic in New York City. These portrayals, while reflecting real professionals, contribute to a limited and homogenous image of veterinarians.[26,27]

"The Vet Life," a reality TV show on Animal Planet, features 3 African-American veterinarians—Dr Diarra Blue, Dr Aubrey Ross, and Dr Michael Lavigne—who run a veterinary practice in Houston, Texas. This show provides a rare representation of Black veterinarians, showcasing their professional and personal lives as they manage their clinic and interact with the community.[28]

Media representation matters because it shapes perceptions, aspirations, and self-identity. When people of color see themselves represented in various professions on screen, it can inspire them to pursue similar paths. Conversely, the absence of BIPOC representation can signal that certain fields are not welcoming or accessible to them.[29]

For individuals from underrepresented groups, seeing successful veterinarians who share their background can provide a sense of possibility and motivation. Role models in media can also offer practical insights into the profession, demystifying the path to becoming a veterinarian.[30]

LANGUAGE ACCESSIBILITY

A 2016 study published in the *Journal of the American Veterinary Medical Association* found that only 8% of responding veterinary practices had staff who could converse in Spanish.[31] This statistic highlights a significant gap in language accessibility within veterinary practices, given that Spanish is the second most spoken language in the United States.[32] While the study did not include data for other languages, representation for other non-English languages is likely even lower.

The implications of this gap in language accessibility are profound. Many pet owners, particularly those from immigrant communities, face challenges in communicating effectively with veterinary staff. This often necessitates the involvement of English-speaking children to act as interpreters during veterinary visits. This practice not only places undue responsibility on the children but also can lead to misunderstandings and compromised care for animal patients.

Furthermore, the lack of linguistic and cultural representation in veterinary practices has broader implications for the field. Children who regularly interpret for their parents in veterinary settings do not see role models who look or speak like them in these professional roles. This lack of representation can deter them from considering careers in veterinary medicine, despite their close interactions with animals.

Addressing language barriers in veterinary practices is crucial for improving service accessibility and ensuring quality care for all animals. Practices should consider hiring bilingual staff and providing training for existing employees in commonly spoken languages. Additionally, translating educational and marketing materials into multiple languages can enhance communication and foster a more inclusive environment, leading to more equitable outcomes.[33]

THE "INTENSIVE PET PARENTING IDEOLOGY"

In the article "Unfit Stewards: The Role of the Intensive Pet Parenting Ideology in Constructing Racialized Narratives," Dr Adilia E.E. James argues that the underrepresentation of people of color in the veterinary profession is partly due to the "intensive pet parenting ideology."[34] This ideology values animals as constant human companions and emphasizes self-sacrificing behaviors including excessive spending and time and lifestyle devotion to pets. This socially constructed ideology is primarily held by wealthy and middle-class White individuals who view their pets as family members.

The author interviewed 44 veterinarians and veterinary students (45% of whom were people of color or multiracial), finding that many believed that to be a veterinarian, one must behave and view animals much like the "intensive pet parent" would. Across race, those interviewed also believed that BIPOC cultures do not promote the pet parenting ideology or prioritize pet care to the same extent as White cultures, and the author rightfully argues this is not supported by academic research. In fact, the AVMA's 2018 *U.S. Pet Ownership and Demographics Sourcebook* confirms that people of all races have very similar familial attitudes toward their cats and dogs.[5] Together, these racialized narratives can lead to assumptions about BIPOC communities and, in particular, BIPOC veterinary professionals, hindering their entry and advancement within the profession and justifying occupational segregation.

James concludes that as a result of the intensive pet parenting ideology, aspiring and graduated veterinary professionals across race have normalized the lack of racial and ethnic diversity in the profession. James points out that when the veterinary world attributes the lack of diversity to a deficit in BIPOC cultures' perceptions of animals, the real reasons for the lack of racial diversity in the profession are obscured and left unaddressed.[34]

DISCRIMINATION AND BIAS

Discrimination and bias can manifest in various ways within veterinary settings, impacting both professionals and clients. For instance, veterinary professionals from BIPOC backgrounds may face microaggressions, overt racism, and exclusionary practices in the workplace. Such experiences can lead to lower job satisfaction, higher stress levels, and ultimately higher turnover rates among these staff members.[35]

Additionally, BIPOC clients may receive subpar care for their animals due to implicit biases held by veterinary staff. This can cause worse health outcomes for their pets and discourage them from seeking veterinary care in the future, which has broader public health implications. For example, diseases that could be prevented or managed with timely veterinary care may go untreated, posing risks to both animal and human health.

The lack of diversity can also affect the client–veterinarian relationship. Research has shown that human patients are more likely to have positive health outcomes, increased health care use, and more affordable treatments when treated by professionals of the same race or ethnicity, a principle that likely extends to veterinary care.[36] While it is not possible or necessary that every client be supported by a veterinary professional of the same race or ethnicity, this underscores the importance of having a racially and ethnically diverse veterinary workforce to ensure all communities receive accessible, high-quality care.

A SNOWBALLING EFFECT

A lack of racial and ethnic diversity in a field like veterinary medicine can have a snowballing effect in several ways.

- Limited role models and mentors: When few people of color are represented in the profession, young people from underrepresented groups may not see themselves reflected in the field. This can discourage them from pursuing veterinary medicine, perpetuating the lack of racial and ethnic diversity.

- Cultural barriers: A lack of diversity can create a culture that may not be welcoming or inclusive to people from different backgrounds. This can make it difficult for underrepresented individuals to feel like they belong, leading to higher employee attrition rates and a further decrease in racial and ethnic diversity.
- Bias in recruitment and retention: A homogenous workforce may unintentionally perpetuate biases in recruitment and retention practices, favoring individuals who fit the existing mold and further excluding those from underrepresented groups.
- Impact on client services: A lack of racial and ethnic diversity among veterinary professionals can create barriers to effective communication and trust with clients from BIPOC backgrounds, potentially impacting the quality of care provided to their animals.

This snowballing effect creates a vicious cycle where the lack of racial and ethnic diversity perpetuates itself, making it increasingly difficult to achieve a more inclusive and representative workforce. For this reason, it is imperative that we actively and urgently confront these issues.

When an issue seems too entrenched and difficult to change, it can be overwhelming and discouraging. Overcoming these barriers requires a multifaceted approach that goes beyond simply hiring a few BIPOC employees or increasing racial representation without implementing the substantive changes that must accompany these initiatives for successful and long-standing outcomes to be achieved. It necessitates a commitment to transforming culture through continuous learning via racial equity education and training to confront one's own biases and how they manifest in veterinary settings, establishing mentorship programs for underrepresented employees, the timely addressing of racial disparities and racial harm in academic institutions and in the workplace, and ensuring equitable opportunities for entry and advancement.

DISCLOSURE

Declaration of artificial intelligence (AI) and AI-assisted technologies in the writing process. During the preparation of this article, the author used ChatGPT4 and Google Gemini in order to improve readability. After using these tools, the author reviewed and edited the content as needed and takes full responsibility for the content of the publication.

REFERENCES

1. U.S. Bureau of Labor Statistics. Labor Force Characteristics by Race and Ethnicity. 2023. Available at: https://www.bls.gov/cps/cpsaat11.htm. [Accessed 21 May 2024].
2. Mattson K. Veterinary educational debt continues to rise. JAVMA News. 2020. Available at: https://www.avma.org/javma-news/2020-12-15/veterinary-educational-debt-continues-rise. [Accessed 28 May 2024].
3. Harper SR, Patton LD, Wooden OS. Access and Equity for African American Students in Higher Education: A Critical Race Historical Analysis of Policy Efforts. J High Educ 2009;80(4):389–414.
4. Boatright K. Veterinary Mental Health and the Influence of Culture. Today's Veterinary Practice. 2022. Available at: https://todaysveterinarypractice.com/veterinary-mental-health-and-the-influence-of-culture. [Accessed 28 May 2024].
5. U.S. Pet Ownership & Demographics Sourcebook. American Veterinary Medical Association. 2018. Available at: https://www.avma.org/resources-tools/reports-statistics/us-pet-ownership-statistics. [Accessed 28 May 2024].

6. Marx MB, Stallones L, Garrity TF, et al. Demographics of pet ownership among U.S. adults 21 to 64 years of age. Anthrozoös 1988;2(1):33–7.
7. Shapiro T, Meschede T, Osoro S. The Roots of the Widening Racial Wealth Gap: Explaining the Black-White Economic Divide. Institute on Assets and Social Policy, Brandeis University, 2013. Available at: https://heller.brandeis.edu/iere/pdfs/racial-wealth-equity/racial-wealth-gap/roots-widening-racial-wealth-gap.pdf. (Accessed 28 May 2024).
8. Rothstein R. The color of lww: a forgotten history of how our government segregated America. New York: Liveright Publishing Corporation; 2018.
9. Kochhar R. and Moslimani M. Wealth gaps across racial and ethnic groups. Pew research center, 2023. Available at: www.pewresearch.org/2023/12/04/wealth-gaps-across-racial-and-ethnic-groups/. (Accessed 28 May 2024).
10. Turner MA, Ross SL, Galster GC, et al. Discrimination in Metropolitan Housing Markets: National Results from Phase I of HDS2000. US Department of Housing and Urban Development. 2002. Available at: https://www.huduser.gov/Publications/pdf/Phase1_Report.pdf. [Accessed 28 May 2024].
11. U.S. Census Bureau. Quarterly Residential Vacancies and Homeownership, Fourth Quarter. 2023. Available at: https://www.census.gov/housing/hvs/current/index.html. [Accessed 30 May 2024].
12. Access to Veterinary Care: Barriers, Current Practices, and Public Policy. Access to Veterinary Care Coalition. 2018. Available at: https://www.avccreport.org. [Accessed 28 May 2024].
13. Urban Institute. Causes and Consequences of Separate and Unequal Neighborhoods. Available at: https://www.urban.org/racial-equity-analytics-lab/structural-racism-explainer-collection/causes-and-consequences-separate-and-unequal-neighborhoods. [Accessed 21 May 2024].
14. American Veterinary Medical Association (AVMA). Financing Your Veterinary Medical Education. AVMA website. Available at: https://www.avma.org/membership/SAVMA/financing-your-veterinary-medical-education. [Accessed 28 May 2024].
15. Association of American Medical Colleges. Tuition and Student Fees Reports. Available at: https://students-residents.aamc.org/media/12846/download. [Accessed 31 May 2024].
16. Bureau of Labor Statistics (BLS). Occupational Outlook Handbook: Veterinarians. 2023. Available at: https://www.bls.gov/ooh/healthcare/veterinarians.htm. [Accessed 28 May 2024].
17. Bureau of Labor Statistics (BLS). Occupational Outlook Handbook: Physicians and Surgeons. 2021. Available at: https://www.bls.gov/ooh/healthcare/physicians-and-surgeons.htm. [Accessed 28 May 2024].
18. U.S. Bureau of Labor Statistics. Veterinary Technologists and Technicians. Available at: https://www.bls.gov/ooh/healthcare/veterinary-technologists-and-technicians.htm. [Accessed 31 May 2024].
19. Hu S, Hood M, Creed PA, et al. The relationship between family socioeconomic status and career outcomes: a life history perspective. J Career Dev 2020; 49(3):493–507.
20. Pew Research Center. Wealth Gaps Rise to Record Highs Between Whites, Blacks, Hispanics. 2011. Available at: https://www.pewresearch.org/social-trends/2011/07/26/wealth-gaps-rise-to-record-highs-between-whites-blacks-hispanics/. [Accessed 28 May 2024].
21. Smith DF. Lessons of history in veterinary medicine. J Vet Med Educ 2013; 40(1):6–11.

22. Strayhorn TL. The absence of African-American Men in Higher Education and Veterinary Medicine. J Vet Med Educ 2009;36(4):351–8.
23. Camus MS, Johnson CM, Sellers G, et al. Auburn is committed to addressing the rural shortage. J Am Vet Med Assoc 2023;261(12).
24. Asare A. The attitudes of minority junior high and high school students toward veterinary medicine. J Vet Med Educ 2011;34(2):47–50.
25. Amass SF. Representations of the veterinary profession in nonfiction children's books. J Am Vet Med Assoc 2011;238(9):1126–30.
26. Nat Geo Wild. Dr Oakley, Yukon Vet. Available at: https://www.nationalgeographic.com/tv/show/84543fcd-ee6a-4f05-a811-1f1b89cd0bdf/about-the-show. [Accessed 28 May 2024].
27. Animal Practice. Available at: https://www.nbc.com/animal-practice. [Accessed 28 May 2024].
28. Animal Planet. The Vet Life. Available at: https://www.animalplanet.com/show/the-vet-life-animal-planet. [Accessed 28 May 2024].
29. Gordon MK. Achievement scripts: Media influences on Black students' academic performance, self-perceptions, and career interests. J Black Psychol 2016;42(3):195–220.
30. Chen Y, So WWM, Zhu J, et al. STEM learning opportunities and career aspirations: The interactive effect of students' self-concept and perceptions of STEM professionals. Int J STEM Educ 2024;11(1):1–21.
31. Landau R, Beck A, Glickman L, et al. Preparedness of small animal veterinary practices to communicate with Spanish-speaking pet owners with limited proficiency in English. J Am Vet Med Assoc 2016;248(6):687–94.
32. U.S. Census Bureau. Language Use in the United States: 2011. Available at: https://www.census.gov/data/tables/2011/demo/2009-lang-tables.html. [Accessed 30 May 2024].
33. Vélez-Contreras R. Breaking the language barrier: The importance of bilingual veterinarians. DVM360. 2023. Available at: https://www.dvm360.com/view/breaking-the-language-barrier-the-importance-of-bilingual-veterinarians. [Accessed 30 May 2024].
34. James AEE. Unfit stewards: the role of the intensive pet parenting ideology in constructing racialized narratives. J Vet Med Educ 2023;50(2):103–10.
35. Mattson K. Veterinary leaders discuss how to combat racism, be an ally. JAVMA News. 2021. Available at: https://www.avma.org/javma-news/2021-02-15/veterinary-leaders-discuss-how-combat-racism-be-ally.
36. Jetty A, Jabbarpour Y, Pollack J, et al. Patient-physician racial concordance associated with improved healthcare use and lower healthcare expenditures in minority populations. J Racial Ethn Health Disparities 2022;9(1):68–81.

Building a Diverse Pipeline

The Current State of Outreach and Engagement Efforts in Veterinary Medicine

Corlice Atkins, JD[a,*], Vernard Hodges, DVM[b,c]

KEYWORDS

• DEI • Diversity in veterinary medicine • Veterinary medicine • Vet for a day

KEY POINTS

- Veterinary medicine is one of the least diverse professions in the United States.
- Approximately 70% of African American veterinarians graduate from the Tuskegee University College of Veterinary Medicine.
- Other veterinary schools and veterinarian-led outreach programs are trying to increase diversity in the profession.

HISTORICAL PERSPECTIVE

The issue of race in America is as old as America itself. African Americans and other minorities in this country were treated differently from and not afforded the same privileges as their White counterparts, and we were consistently subjected to legal discrimination until recent history. Although African Americans have been in the United States since the founding of this country, we have had to fight for the right to be considered actual people, to become citizens, to use the same facilities as White people, and to attend the same schools as White people.

Not only were African Americans subjected to legal discrimination and subjected to slavery for hundreds of years, we were not even seen as actual human beings. During the Constitutional Convention, it was determined that African Americans were only three-fifths of a person; 3 out of 5 slaves were counted for population purposes.[1] The highest Court of the land decreed in the *Dred Scott* decision that African Americans were not citizens,[2] the prevailing law until the ratification of the 14th Amendment. While universities were being established in America, African Americans were still

[a] Vet for a Day, Bonaire, GA, USA; [b] 102 Starlight Drive, Bonaire, GA 31005, USA; [c] Critter Fixer Veterinary Hospital, Warner Robins, GA, USA

* Corresponding author. 1217 S. Houston Lake Road, Suite 2, Warner Robins, GA 31088, USA.

E-mail address: catkins@atkinslawllc.com

Twitter: @drhodges (V.H.)

Vet Clin Small Anim 54 (2024) 767–776

https://doi.org/10.1016/j.cvsm.2024.06.001 vetsmall.theclinics.com

enslaved on plantations and forbidden to learn how to read. The Supreme Court again ruled to enforce egregious discriminatory practices sanctioned by state and federal governments in *Plessy v Ferguson*, holding that segregation was legal by providing separate facilities for the races, as long as they were equal.

Of course, in the era of Jim Crow, legislatures and courts were not enforcing the equality side of the separate but equal doctrine, leaning instead on ensuring that African Americans were kept separate from White people. The separate but equal rule was especially harsh in the Deep South, where racial tensions had run high since the birth of the nation. Facilities for African Americans were often underfunded and kept in deplorable conditions. Not until the NAACP, led by legal giant Thurgood Marshall, challenged the separate equal doctrine through *Brown v Board of Education* and its companion cases with its argument that *Plessy* was unconstitutional, violating the 14th Amendment, which guarantees that states shall not deny any person within their jurisdiction equal protection of the laws.

Brown, which was decided in 1954, paved the way for school desegregation. Naturally, schools and governing bodies that had embraced segregation for such a long time were resistant to change, even when the order for change came from the Supreme Court of the United States. The University of Alabama did not admit African American students until 1963, almost 10 years after school desegregation was ruled unlawful, and then it was only done with the intervention of the courts and federal authorities. Shockingly, there is a school district in Cleveland, Mississippi, that did not desegregate until 2016, when a District Court Judge ordered the town to combine 2 segregated high schools into 1 integrated school[3]; prior to the issuance of this order, the high school on one side of the railroad tracks remained 99.7% African American despite a 50 year legal battle in which the federal government repeatedly instructed the town to integrate the schools.

During slavery and Reconstruction, the Black church, forward-thinking African Americans and White people sympathetic to our cause founded a number of what are now known as historically Black colleges or universities (HBCUs). HBCUs were created as a direct response to the racial discrimination that kept African Americans out of established schools and universities. The earliest HBCUs taught mostly agriculture, education, and theology to produce educated farmers, teachers, and preachers,[4] but eventually they branched out to educate African Americans in every field imaginable. Even after school desegregation, HBCUs continued to thrive, partially because they created safe spaces for African American students to learn and grow[5] without the threat of racial animus.

Agricultural careers have been particularly affected by America's racist past. The Great Migration occurred when millions of African Americans fled the oppressive South with hopes of more job opportunities and better living conditions in the Northern cities. Not only were they leaving their homes, but they were also leaving their friends, their churches, and sometimes their family members behind.[6] Additionally, they were leaving their way of life, going from rural settings to cramped, crowded city life that required a different set of skills. The Great Migration may well have contributed to the decline of interest among African Americans in the agricultural and veterinary fields.

According to the Pew Research Center, in 2022, African Americans made up 14.4% of the population of the United States.[7] Despite our contribution to this nation and our storied history and accomplishments, we fail to be accurately represented in certain professions, none more so than veterinary medicine. For instance, 5.7% of medical doctors are African American[8] and 4.7% of attorneys are African American,[9] but only 2.2% of veterinarians are African American,[10] and that statistical remains woefully stagnant.

The first African American doctor to graduate from an American medical school—David J. Peck—earned his medical degree (MD) from Rush Medical College in 1847.[11] The first medical school at an HBCU, the Howard University College of Medicine, was founded in 1868,[12] less than 20 years after Dr Peck earned his degree. The first African American person to earn a law degree from an American university was George Lewis Ruffin, who graduated from Harvard Law School in 1869.[13] The Howard University School of Law was founded in 1869, the same year as Ruffin's graduation.[14]

More than 20 years after, the first Doctor of Veterinary Medicine (DVM) degree was conferred in the United States to Dr Daniel Salmon[15] by Cornell University in 1876; the first recorded African American veterinarian—Dr Augustus Nathaniel Lushington[16]—earned his DVM from the University of Pennsylvania in 1897. Although he faced prejudice, Dr Lushington established a large animal practice in rural Virginia.

It is important to note the period between the first African American graduate in the field and the founding of a corresponding professional school at an HBCU. Less than 20 years passed between the time of David Beck's earning his MD and the establishment of the Howard University College of Medicine, and that time span was even shorter between George Lewis Ruffin's earning a Juris Doctor and the establishment of the Howard University School of Law—less than a year.

Conversely, the first veterinary school at an HBCU, now referred to as the Tuskegee University College of Veterinary Medicine (TUCVM), was founded in 1945, almost 50 years after Dr Lushington graduated from Cornell. Prior to the inception of TUCVM, there were only 70 African Americans [17] reported to have earned DVM degrees. African Americans interested in veterinary medicine were at a disadvantage to their peers who wanted to pursue medical or law degrees. Those individuals had HBCUs that welcomed them with open arms, while prior to TUCVM's founding, prospective veterinarians could only hope that they would be admitted to schools with histories of racial segregation.

Since the founding of TUCVM, they have graduated over 3000 veterinarians, and almost 75% of Black veterinarians have matriculated there.[18] While we do not have hard data on the total number of African American veterinarians who have graduated from TUCVM, we can safely say that number is in the thousands. If we contrast 70 veterinarians in 50 years to thousands of veterinarians in 70 years, we can see the effect an HBCU degree program has on the Black population in that field.

While TUCVM has graduated the overwhelming majority of African American veterinarians, other veterinary schools are making strides to address the lack of diversity in the profession. HBCUs have assumed the responsibility of ensuring that higher education is available to minorities, but it is not a burden they should have to bear alone.

CURRENT PIPELINE

Diversity Initiatives

Diversity is important in veterinary medicine for several reasons: a diverse population is best suited to serve a diverse clientele and increased diversity results in different perspectives and better outcomes. It will take significant sustained work from the veterinary community to combat the history of institutional racism that has contributed to a lack of diversity in the veterinary profession, but there are many who are committed to doing the work to change those statistics.

Several veterinary schools have established initiatives to combat the low number of minorities in veterinary medicine. Many schools have also established positions or offices dedicated to diversity, equity, and inclusion (DEI) efforts. These schools are to be commended for recognizing the issues and working to help resolve them. For example, the University of Georgia College in veterinary medicine formed a DEI Office in 2020, and the school has a voluntary certificate in Diversity and Inclusion program, a speaker series, and an anti-racism course.[19] The Ohio State University College of Veterinary Medicine has put into place recruitment efforts for students from kindergarten through undergraduates that have touched over 10,000 students.[20] Under Dean Rustin Moore's leadership, the Ohio State University College of Veterinary Medicine has increased the number of minority students from 13% of the class in 2018 to 36% of the class in 2024.[20]

The Auburn University College of Veterinary Medicine has a strategic plan that calls for attracting a diverse student population by hiring a recruitment and diversity officer; increasing outreach activities for students in rural communities and cities; and engaging at least one underrepresented group each month.[21]

The University of California Davis School of Veterinary Medicine (UCSVM) is a shining example of a veterinary school leaning in and focusing on increasing diversity. They appointed their first Chief Diversity Officer to oversee diversity initiatives. They have recruitment scholarships for underrepresented minority populations.[22]

UCSVM has specific efforts for students beginning at the elementary level; they have an afterschool program for children in grades kindergarten through fourth that was created by the Purdue College of Veterinary Medicine called This is How We Role.[23] This is How We Role is a program where veterinary professionals help young children who are educationally disadvantaged due to socioeconomic status, race, or ethnicity learn about careers in veterinary medicine. The goal is to diversify veterinary medicine by taking the information to the kids and starting early.

UCSVM has a 5 week residential program for high-achieving, underrepresented minority high school students from the Sacramento area in 9th through 11th grade called SMASH. SMASH focuses on not only developing skills but also focuses on developing networks, building relationships, and building confidence.[24] UCSVM also has the Vet Med Exploration Academy, a 3 day academy held each fall that gives underrepresented students a first-hand look at the fields of study that make up a veterinary medical education.[22]

For undergraduate students, UCSVM has the Summer Enrichment Program,[25] an intensive 4 week program to help disadvantaged, low-income, or historically underrepresented students enhance their preparation for veterinary school. The Summer Enrichment Program began over 30 years ago and consists of clinical rotations, field trips, lectures, presentations, and workshops. Costs are covered based on need and availability, and students receive a stipend, which is important to students who are economically disadvantaged.

UCSVM notes that since they are the only public DVM program in the state of California, "it is [their] responsibility to serve the citizens of the state of California and to reflect the demographics of the state population in [their] student population."[26] UCSVM has made extraordinary strides in maintaining a diverse population: almost 50% of the student body is made up of minorities. They have instituted implicit bias and cultural humility training.[27]

Another example of a veterinary school making a strong commitment to DEI is the Purdue University College of Veterinary Medicine (PUCVM). Dean Willie Reed, who earned his undergraduate degree and DVM from Tuskegee University and his PhD from Purdue University,[28] was appointed to lead the school in 2007, and in 2008, the Office of Diversity and Inclusion (now known as the Office of Diversity, Equity and Inclusion) was established. In 2012, PUCVM implemented their first diversity strategic plan, and the following year, they established the Center for Excellence in Diversity and Inclusion in partnership with the AAVMC and the AVMA.[29]

PUCVM's current DEI plan has strategic goals to, among other things, integrate diversity, equity, and inclusion into the academic principles of teaching, research, and engagement and recruit and advance a diverse community of faculty, staff, and students.[29] Like UCSVM, PUCVM has a framework of innovative programming that is aimed to reach students from high school to college. The PUCVM program, launched in 2019, is called Vet Up. Vet Up Champions is a cohort of 26 individuals, ranging from rising high school juniors to second-year undergraduate students.[30] Nontraditional learners are also eligible to join. The year-long program prepares participants for veterinary school by mentorship, finance and cultural competence training, and exposure to different career paths.

The Vet Up College program is a 6 week residential summer program for 26 educationally or economically disadvantaged undergraduates who are from underrepresented minority groups; from rural backgrounds; first-generation college students; or from low-income households that prepares students to be competitive in the DVM applicant pool.[31] The Vet Up College program mimics the actual DVM curriculum, as well as educating students on issues impacting the veterinary profession. The program also educates participants on the competitive application and admissions process. Participants who meet a number of criteria will also be invited to apply to the Vet Up College Early Admissions program, which has a selection approach that considers both academic and nonacademic factors.

Those students selected to the early admissions program are not left to fend for themselves. They are known as Vet Up DVM scholars, and they have daily structured group study sessions, a professional focus profile that helps them identify and learn how to reach their desired career goals and meetings each semester with professors to determine how they can perform better.[32] The Vet Up program is a structured wraparound program that works to guarantee the success of those who participate.

PUCVM also encourages those outside their community to learn and grow in the DEI space. Their certificate for Diversity & Inclusion in Veterinary Medicine[33] is open to all members of the veterinary medical community, including academic administration, faculty, staff, and students, and practicing veterinary medical professionals. The certificate is comprehensive, covering areas from the history of diversity in veterinary medicine to microaggressions to leadership. PUCVM's willingness to share their well-crafted course with those outside the schools evidences their commitment to educate everyone, which is key to solving the issue of lack of diversity.

There are also many veterinarian-led programs aimed at increasing awareness of the veterinary profession among underserved populations. Veterinarians nationwide are visiting classes, attending career days, hosting students in their clinics, providing individual mentorship, hosting camps, and spreading the word using all of their resources.

At Critter Fixer Veterinary Hospital, we have used our resources to start a youth program called Critter Fixer Vet for a Day. In 2020, Nat Geo Wild aired the first season of "Critter Fixers: Country Vets," a docuseries about 2 African American men, Drs Terrence Ferguson and Vernard Hodges, practicing veterinary medicine in rural Georgia. After the success of the show, the clinics were inundated with calls, emails, and letters from viewers. The show marked the first appearance of African American veterinarians on Nat Geo Wild, and as the seasons progressed, the 2 main items people communicated were (1) they had never seen a Black veterinarian and (2) they had no idea how the young people in their lives could pursue a career in veterinary medicine.

When the television show aired, there was no way to know it would serve as a pipeline for more minorities to learn about veterinary medicine. We found, based on anecdotal evidence, that African American students were not exploring veterinary medicine because of a lack of awareness and opportunity. Only 34% of African American adults are pet owners as compared to 68% of White adults.[34] Therefore, fewer African American children grow up with pets in the home and thus did not need services of a veterinarian. Since some African American children had never seen African American veterinarians, they did not consider veterinary medicine as a career choice. Studies have shown that children choose careers based on the careers of their close family members,[35] so the lack of African American veterinarians and pet owners directly impacts the number of African American children who choose veterinary medicine as a career option.

Once African Americans become aware of the veterinary profession, they are far behind their White peers who have grown up seeing White veterinarians, both personally and professionally. The AAVMC reports that applicants to the class of 2027 reported a mean of 1860 hours[36] of experiential hours in a veterinary setting. A minority student just learning that a career in veterinary medicine is possible during her undergraduate career would have an almost insurmountable goal to be competitive with her peers. A high school or college student first must find a veterinary setting that allows him to obtain those crucial experiential hours and then find the time to complete the hours. As we mentioned earlier, many African American students do not know any veterinarians, so that is a barrier to their ability to obtain the requisite hours to apply for veterinary school.

Critter Fixer Veterinary Hospital is located 15 minutes away from Fort Valley State University, the alma mater of both Drs Hodges and Ferguson. Fort Valley State University, an HBCU, has the only American Veterinary Medical Association accredited 4 year veterinary technology program in the state of Georgia.[37] As such, we have a unique opportunity to foster interest locally in the veterinary sciences. We have a constant flow of young people in the clinics getting prepared for the arduous task of applying for veterinary school. Critter Fixer Vet for a Day was born from requests coming in from across the country to provide assistance to those outside the Middle Georgia region.

Having worked with young people for many years, Critter Fixer Vet for a Day recognized the issues of awareness and accessibility, and we built the program to give as many children as possible the best opportunity we could to be successful in the veterinary field. We strive to expose children to the profession at a young age—between 12 and 16 years. We want to get young people excited about the profession and about the possibilities that lie ahead. Reaching students in middle school and early high school gives students and their families time to explore higher education and volunteer opportunities. A key component of Critter Fixer Vet for a Day is to match participants with mentors in their local area, thereby helping them remain interested and engaged and helping them acquire the hours needed to apply for vet school. Another aim of the program is to get the veterinary community involved and invested in helping to bridge the gap.

We have received tremendous support from industry leaders, like the Zoetis Foundation, the Hill's Pet Nutrition, and the PetSmart Veterinary Services, and buy-in from the American Veterinary Medical Association. With the support of our partners, we have been able to move almost 1000 young people through Critter Fixer Vet for a Day and match close to 50 with local mentors or shadowing opportunities. We have also partnered with the National Association for Black Veterinarian (NABV), bringing members from their student chapters as ambassadors to our programs to assist young people in undergraduate pre-veterinary programs find internships that will bolster their veterinary school applications.

The goal of NABV is to create a pipeline into veterinary medicine for African Americans.[38] NABV, and organizations like it, provides networking and mentoring opportunities, connecting students with professionals. This grassroots approach gives students opportunities to shadow and intern and to make connections with veterinarians who can write recommendation letters and potentially provide employment opportunities or suggestions.

FUTURE GOALS

There is no doubt that there is an upcoming shortage of veterinarians. A study commissioned by Mars indicates that by 2030, up to 55,000 additional veterinarians will be required to meet the needs of the number of companion animals.[39] The veterinary community has responded in a major way; there are over a dozen prospective veterinary schools either in the planning stages or with classes scheduled to begin.[40] There are currently only 32 operational veterinary schools in the United States, compared to 192 medical schools[41] and 197 law schools.[42] Certainly, increasing the number of schools increases the number of seats available and will afford greater opportunities for a more diverse veterinary population.

New Historically Black College or University Vet School

Among the new planned veterinary schools, one will be located at the University of Maryland Eastern Shore (UMES),[43] an HBCU. The school which is scheduled to accept students in fall 2026. This vet school will be only the second veterinary school at an HBCU. The Founding Dean of the UMES Veterinary School, Dr Kimberly Braxton, believes that the addition of another HBCU vet school "will of course attract the attention of students interested in the profession, which will then influence more HBCUs to take notice and follow in our footsteps. Developing this school with consistency, continuity, and quality and adding a second HBCU veterinary school will be a positive influence for the pipeline of minorities to the veterinary profession." The President of UMES, Dr Heidi Anderson, believes that the school will "increase both the diversity of the profession and address the workforce needs of the industry."[44] The Dean of the UMES School of Agriculture and Natural Sciences, Moses Kairo, says they will aim to graduate 100 students per year, and the school also plans to graduate students in 3 years instead of the tradition 4 years by using student time "more effectively."

Reflecting on the increase of African American veterinarians with the founding of TUCVM makes us hopeful that the additional HBCU veterinary school will exponentially increase the number of African American veterinarians, but it will also create a natural pipeline from other HBCUs, who will certainly take notice and funnel students to UMES.

SUMMARY

There are many reasons the minority population is so low in veterinary medicine, but none as compelling as the aftereffects of school segregation. African Americans were legally barred from attending the same schools as their White counterparts and thus were not afforded the same opportunities. The separate but equal doctrine was a farce; the overwhelming majority of African Americans did not have access to a veterinary school that would allow their entry.

The establishment of the TUCVM changed the game. It opened the floodgates for African Americans to pursue veterinary medicine, but we had a lot of catching up to do. Schools like UC Davis School of Veterinary Medicine and the PUCVM had been working diligently, both in the forefront and behind the scenes, and most other veterinary schools have joined the fight.

Programs and organizations that exist separate and apart from veterinary schools have also been putting forth efforts to perform outreach and education and create interest and opportunities for minority students interested in veterinary medicine, and with proper funding and support, these programs can make a true difference in supporting the pipeline to veterinary school for minorities.

The large number of veterinary schools on the horizon, especially with the addition of another HBCU veterinary school, bodes well for an increase in the number of minorities who will be able to attend. Outreach and engagement for minority students will not only help diversify the profession, but it will help combat the veterinary shortage. The inclusion of minorities in the profession will be a positive for all.

DISCLOSURE

The authors have nothing to disclose.

REFERENCES

1. The three-fifths compromise, perspectives of change. Available at: https://perspectivesofchange.hms.harvard.edu/node/87#:~:text=TheThree%2DFifths Compromisewas,forlegislativerepresentationandtaxation. Accessed December 12, 2023.
2. Dred Scott vs Sandford (1857), Milestone documents. Available at: https://www.archives.gov/milestone-documents/dred-scott-v-sandford#:~:text=Inthisruling%2CtheU.S.,slaveryfromaFederalterritory. Accessed December 12, 2023.
3. Domonoske C. After 50-Year Legal Struggle, Mississippi school district ordered to desegregate, NPR. Available at: https://www.npr.org/sections/thetwo-way/2016/05/17/478389720/after-50-year-legal-struggle-mississippi-school-district-ordered-to-desegregate. Accessed December 13, 2023.
4. The history of HBCUs in America, APM Reports. Available at: https://www.apmreports.org/episode/2015/08/20/the-history-of-hbcus-in-america. Accessed December 13, 2023.
5. Atkins, Howard University, B.A., 2001, Howard University School of Law, J.D., 2004; Hodges, Fort Valley State University, B.S., 1993, Tuskegee University College of Veterinary Medicine DVM, 1997.
6. Long Lasting Legacy, Great migration, smithsonian magazine. Available at: https://www.smithsonianmag.com/history/long-lasting-legacy-great-migration-180960118/. Accessed December 15, 2023.
7. Facts about the US Black Population, Pew Research Center. Available at: https://www.pewresearch.org/social-trends/fact-sheet/facts-about-the-us-black-population/. Accessed December 7, 2023.
8. National Medical Association. Only 5.7% of US doctors are Black, and experts warn the shortage harms public health. Available at: https://www.nmanet.org/news/632592/Only-5.7-of-US-doctors-are-Black-and-experts-warn-the-shortage-harms-public-health.htm#:~:text=XEmailLinkedIn-,Only5.7%25ofUSdoctorsareBlack%2Candexpertswarn,theshortageharmspublichealth. Accessed December 7, 2023.
9. ABA Survey finds 1.3 M lawyers in the US, American Bar Association. Available at: https://www.americanbar.org/news/abanews/aba-news-archives/2022/06/aba-lawyers-survey/. Accessed December 12, 2023.
10. Being Black in a White Profession- closing the gap on racial representation, RUSVM Blog. Available at: https://veterinary.rossu.edu/about/blog/closing-the-gap-on-racial-representation. Accessed December 7, 2023.

11. Celebrating Black history month: reflections on the legacy of David Jones Peck, MD, RUSH stories. Available at: https://www.rush.edu/news/celebrating-black-history-month-reflections-legacy-david-jones-peck-md. Accessed December 2, 2023.
12. History, Howard University. Available at: https://medicine.howard.edu/about/history. Accessed December 2, 2023.
13. Key Events in Black Higher Education, JBHE. Available at: https://jbhe.com/chronology/#:~:text=1869: AGeorgeLewisRuffinis,'firstAfrican - DAmericanjudge. Accessed December 2, 2023.
14. History, School of Law, Howard University. Available at: https://law.howard.edu/about/our-history. Accessed December 13, 2023.
15. LEGENDS: America's first DVM, AVMA. Available at: https://www.avma.org/javma-news/2013-03-01/legends-americas-first-dvm#:~:text=Dr.-,DanielE.,undertheleadershipofDr. Accessed December 2, 2023.
16. Black History Month in Animal Welfare – Dr Augustus Nathaniel Lushington, Michigan Humane. Available at: https://www.michiganhumane.org/black-history-month-in-animal-welfare-dr-augustus-nathaniel-lushington/. Accessed December 2, 2023.
17. Adams E. A Historical Overview of African American Veterinarians in the United States: 1889–2000. Available at: https://www.vet.k-state.edu/docs/about/diversity/AA_409.pdf.
18. The Tuskegee University College of Veterinary Medicine Historical Legacy. Available at: https://www.tuskegee.edu/programs-courses/colleges-schools/cvm/cvm-college-of-veterinary-medicine-historical-legacy#:~:text=PattersonfoundedtheUnitedNegro,tostudyveterinarymedicinedue. Accessed December 2, 2023.
19. Diversity and Inclusion at the CVM, University of Georgia. Available at: https://vet.uga.edu/about-us/diversity-and-inclusion/. Accessed December 18, 2023.
20. Progress along our Journey, The Ohio State University. Available at: https://vet.osu.edu/about-college/commitment-diversity-equity-inclusion-and-belonging/progress-along-our-journey. Accessed December 18, 2023.
21. Strategic Plan 2021-2026, Auburn University. Available at: https://www.vetmed.auburn.edu/strategic-plan/strategic-plan-2021-2026/#goal-5. Accessed December 18, 2023.
22. Pre-Vet Outreach and Recruitment, UCDavis veterinary Medicine. Available at: https://www.vetmed.ucdavis.edu/index.php/student-life/diversity/pre-vet-outreach-and-recruitment. Accessed December 18, 2023.
23. How We Role, Purdue University. Available at: https://vet.purdue.edu/engagement/how-we-role/index.php. Accessed December 18, 2023.
24. SMASH Academy. Available at: https://www.smash.org/programs/smash-academy/. Accessed December 18, 2023.
25. Summer Enrichment Program, UC Davis Veterinary Medicine. Available at: https://www.vetmed.ucdavis.edu/admissions/so-you-want-be-veterinarian/summer-enrichment-program. Accessed December 18, 2023.
26. Student University Data, UC Davis Veterinary Medicine. Available at: https://www.vetmed.ucdavis.edu/student-life/diversity/student-diversity-data. Accessed December 18, 2023.
27. Diversity and Inclusion Education, UC Davis Veterinary Medicine. Available at: https://www.vetmed.ucdavis.edu/student-life/diversity/diversity-and-inclusion-education. Accessed December 18, 2023.
28. Office of the Dean, Purdue University. Available at: https://vet.purdue.edu/about/our-people/office-of-the-dean.php. Accessed December 18, 2023.

29. Strategic Plan, Purdue University. Available at: https://vet.purdue.edu/diversity/strategic-plan.php. Accessed December 18, 2023.
30. Vet Up! Champions, Purdue University. Available at: https://vet.purdue.edu/diversity/vetup/champions.php. Accessed December 18, 2023.
31. Vet Up! College program, Purdue University. Available at: https://vet.purdue.edu/diversity/vetup/college.php. Accessed December 18, 2023.
32. Vet Up! DVM Scholars program, Purdue University. Available at: https://vet.purdue.edu/diversity/vetup/scholars.php. Accessed December 18, 2023.
33. Diversity Certificate, Purdue University. Available at: https://vet.purdue.edu/diversity/certificate/. Accessed December 18, 2023.
34. About Half of us Pet Owners say their pets are as much a part of their family as a human member, Pew Research. Available at: https://www.pewresearch.org/short-reads/2023/07/07/about-half-us-of-pet-owners-say-their-pets-are-as-much-a-part-of-their-family-as-a-human-member/sr_2023-07-07_pets_3/. Accessed December 19, 2023.
35. Taking over the family business: children tend to make career choices based on what jobs their parents and siblings have, daily mail online. Available at: https://www.dailymail.co.uk/sciencetech/article-3504404/Taking-family-business-Children-tend-make-career-choices-based-jobs-parents-siblings-have.html. Accessed December 19, 2023.
36. Public Data, American Association of Veterinary Medical Colleges. Available at: https://www.aavmc.org/about-aavmc/public-data/. Accessed December 19, 2023.
37. Veterinary Science and Public Heath. FVSUag. Available at: https://ag.fvsu.edu/departments/veterinary-science-and-public-health. Accessed December 18, 2023.
38. Founders page, National Association for Black Veterinarians. Available at: https://nabvonline.org/founders-page/. Accessed December 17, 2023.
39. Tackling the Veterinary Professional Shortage, MARS Veterinary Health. Available at: https://www.marsveterinary.com/tackling-the-veterinary-professional-shortage/. Accessed December 17, 2023.
40. A proliferation of newly proposed veterinary colleges, AVMA News. Available at: https://www.avma.org/news/proliferation-newly-proposed-veterinary-colleges. Accessed December 17, 2023.
41. How Many Medical Schools in US: The Definitive Guide (2024), International Medical Aid. Available at: https://medicalaid.org/how-many-medical-schools-in-us-the-definitive-guide-2023/#:~:text=HowManyMedicalSchoolsintheUS%3F,States%2Ctotaling192medicalschools. Accessed December 17, 2023.
42. ABA Approved Law Schools, American Bar Association. Available at: https://www.americanbar.org/groups/legal_education/resources/aba_approved_law_schools/. Accessed December 17, 2023.
43. UMES responds to national vet shortage with new School, University of Maryland Eastern Shore. Available at: https://wwwcp.umes.edu/sans/sans-monthly-digest/umes-responds-to-national-vet-shortage-with-new-school/#:~:text=TheUniversitySystemofMaryland,Maryland'sfirststand%2Daloneprogram. Accessed December 17, 2023.
44. UMES vet school could be a first for Maryland and public HBCUs, University of Maryland Eastern Shore. Available at: https://wwwcp.umes.edu/sans/sans-monthly-digest/umes-vet-school-will-be-a-first-for-maryland-and-public-hbcus/. Accessed December 17, 2023.

Diversity, Equity, Inclusion, and Belonging in Veterinary Education

Susan M. Williams, DVM, PhD, ACPV*

KEYWORDS

• Diversity • Equity and inclusion • Disabilities • Communication • Well-being
• Standards for accreditation • Extracurricular events • Affinity groups

KEY POINTS

- Diversity, equity, and inclusion (DEI) is interwoven into accreditation standards.
- Accommodations for students with visible and nonvisible disabilities are important for student success in the professional curriculum and high stakes testing situations.
- Affinity groups can provide support and educational opportunities for students as extracurricular or co-curricular events.
- Communication skills are very important to practice with a diversity of clients.
- Providing an inclusive environment is the responsibility of everyone involved in veterinary medical education and the profession as a whole.

INTRODUCTION

Veterinary education is undergoing changes due to updates in the American Association Veterinary Medical Association's (AAVMA's) Council on Education (COE) accreditation standards.[1] Those changes were approved in July 2022 that interweave diversity, equity, and inclusion (DEI) in several standards versus having a single standard that was diversity centered. These changes have included how to communicate with a diversity of clients with cultural humility, collaboration with a diverse workforce, supporting DEI awareness programs for students, disability or accessibility services for students, recruitment and admission practices, and others. With the requirement to review and update curriculum every 7 years at minimum, many institutions have looked to different curricular methods to incorporate the updated standards into their educational programming. AAVMC created a framework for veterinary education based off the human medicine competency education and named it Competency-Based

Department of Population Health, Poultry Diagnostic and Research Center, College of Veterinary Medicine, University of Georgia, 953 College Station Road, Athens, GA 30602, USA
* Corresponding author.
E-mail address: smwillia@uga.edu

Vet Clin Small Anim 54 (2024) 777–784
https://doi.org/10.1016/j.cvsm.2024.06.002 vetsmall.theclinics.com

Veterinary Education (CBVE) in 2018 that has 9 Domains of Competence.[2] These 9 domains contain a list of competencies that are essential to the veterinary curriculum. There are also examples of subcompetencies that each school can modify that illustrate how to assess whether a competency is met or not by students in the program. These domains can be linked back to COE standards for accreditation purposes. This chapter will review ways DEI concepts are interwoven in Veterinary Medical Education or bring to light where challenges may develop when updating and implementing curriculum. It will also highlight how DEI activities and programming can create a more welcoming environment in the college and eventually the profession.

Here is an overview of the COE standards and where DEI has been interwoven.

Standard 1 Organization

The COE identifies how DEI should be in the accredited college of veterinary medicine by creating a structure and climate that does not discriminate and promote DEI that is consistent with the applicable laws. The standard states that a college "must have and follow a statement on diversity, equity, and inclusion, consistent with applicable law".[1] This may be in the mission statement or a separate statement depending on the institution. By creating expectations around a welcoming and inclusive environment for everyone involved in veterinary education, the leader of the college can really set the tone and promote DEIB (diversity, equity, inclusion and belonging) in everything the college does.

Standard 3 Physical Facilities and Equipment

Most people do not consider how facilities fit into DEIB unless you are that person who it affects directly. The American Disabilities Act demands accessibility for buildings, parking, bathrooms, and so forth for physical disabilities, which most non-physically challenged people also take advantage of by using an elevator, curb cuts in the sidewalks, and larger bathroom stalls for wheelchairs. This means that classrooms, seminar rooms, ambulatory or field services trucks, and so forth need to be accessible for all types of people. Classroom seating is always a challenge, especially in stadium seating spaces or auditoriums. Chairs and desks should be accessible for everyone involved regardless of body type, for example, being over 6 feet tall, left-handed, or mobility issue. Most, if not all, universities have a Disability Resource Center, which has employees that are well-versed in what kinds of furniture are more accommodating. However, sometimes their services are not used prior to planning and renovations and then problems arise when a student, faculty, or staff member needs accessible furniture in a classroom, office, rounds room, conference rooms, or availability of a university vehicle that can accommodate a motorized wheel chair or scooter. It also may become noticeable in surgery suites, radiology spaces, and animal wards where a table may not be adjustable or wide enough work areas to accommodate students or employees with physical limitations. Other facilities that can limit the feeling of belonging are bathrooms. Having gender neutral bathrooms that are easy to find, not only affect students, faculty, and staff of the college, but clients that are transgender feel more welcome. The key is easy to locate, not an afterthought of converting 1 bathroom in a multistory building that become difficult to access. Same can be said for changing rooms and locker rooms.

Standard 6 Students

This standard applies to students that are already in the curriculum. Support services for students must include well-being, academic and personal challenges, learning or other disabilities and diversity, equity, and inclusion awareness programs for students. This is the area where most colleges have some type of affinity group for students. For many years, it was VOICE (currently known as Veterinarians as One Inclusive Community for Empowerment) and Broad Spectrum (now Student Pride VMC). However, many newer affinity groups have started up on campus from student chapters of the National Association for Black Veterinarians (NABV), Association of Asian Veterinary Medical Professionals, and Latinx Veterinary Medical Association along with other national groups like Natives in Vet Med. These groups serve multiple purposes: providing support of individuals with those identities[3–5] and serving as a source of information for the college on issues that affect those groups via educational programming. Some colleges have all of the affinity groups while others have VOICE and Student Pride VMC as the only groups, depending on numbers of historically marginalized students. Most of the newer affinity groups have a national group or organization with veterinary professionals as members of their sponsoring entity. For VOICE, AAVMC is the national organization sponsor.

Other support services that students may need are accommodations for various visible and invisible disabilities. Students have to initiate the accommodation process and provide necessary documentation to support the diagnosis. Once that is completed, accommodations can be made usually via the office of Academic Affairs or similar office to inform faculty of the needs of the student. Universal design is helpful with this by using various teaching methods for those who are auditory learners, visual learners, tactile learners, and so forth. Using PowerPoints with appropriate colors and fonts help everyone and especially those with visual impairments. Having seating that allows students to best see the screens or hear the lecturer is also important when designing or redesigning classroom spaces. Using closed captioning on videos shown in class for those who have auditory processing impairments, having extra time or quiet spaces to take examinations are examples of common accommodations. Having accommodations can provide students the opportunities to do well academically. Not having the accommodations, especially in high stakes testing situations can result in not passing national board examinations or dismissal from programs. An example of this type of result is documented in the Petersen and colleagues paper in 2022 with medical students and United States Medical Licensing Examination Step-1 examination and denial of accommodations.[6] Two hundred seventy six students applied for accommodations and just over half, 144, were denied. 110/144 took the examination without accommodations and 35/110 failed and 4/110 withdrew or were dismissed from the medical program. 74/114 of those denied accommodations, were delayed entry into the next phase of the curriculum. A similar review for dental students was performed and published by Johnson[7] in 2006. Here, the author examined accommodations for the National Board Dental Examination, part I and II along with state or regional licensing tests over a 5-year period. Very small percentage of students requested accommodations and about half were granted. However, some of the agencies did not keep such information or did not release the information due to confidentiality concerns for accommodated test takers.

Because the veterinary college is responsible for promoting an institutional climate and culture that fosters diversity and inclusion, some college may have a more difficult time due to recently passed legislation in the states where they are that limit DEI in some form or matter. They may withhold state funding for DEI offices on campuses or positions that support DEI in the colleges.[8]

Well-being also falls under this Standard. Having counselors available for students can run the gamut from being embedded at the college to having specific counselors at the University support students in the Doctor of Veterinary Medicine curriculum. The lack of multicultural counselors is a concern for students who want to speak with a person that understands what it is like to be a historically marginalized person and all the issues that may come out during their schooling.[4] Anecdotally, students indicated that they do not want to speak with a white counselor or that pressures from their own community prevent them from seeking help when needed.

Standard 7 Admission

This standard has taken a hit with the recent Supreme Court ruling on Affirmative Action for admissions with the 2 cases, Harvard and UNC.[9,10] The standard has been updated to reflect being consistent with applicable laws. Training for admissions committee for bias has also come under attack in some states that prevents mandatory DEI training for faculty.[8] Pipeline programs for recruitment may also have to adjust their recruitment priorities so that race or ethnicity is downplayed in the selection process depending on the state. For example, perhaps they expand recruitment in rural communities or lower socioeconomic areas that have historically marginalized communities present. Opening recruitment to other groups like first generation students, students with disabilities, visible or not visible, or neurodivergent students can still draw populations into veterinary medicine that were not exposed before.

Standard 9 Curriculum

The curriculum part where DEI occurs in section g: "Opportunities throughout the curriculum for students to gain an understanding of the importance influences of DEI in veterinary medicine, including the impact of implicit bias related to an individual's personal circumstances on the delivery of veterinary medical services." How this is done typically falls into the professional skills portion of the curriculum. From simulated client interactions[11,12] to experiential learning opportunities,[13–15] each institution determines how to implement the concepts and teaching strategies. One institution developed a selective course option to explore various DEI topics within the context of veterinary medicine.[16]

Communications training within the curriculum has been more emphasized[17] with various modalities to teach and have students practice communication skills. Example methods include simulated clients, videotape, small groups, and feedback and facilitation skills.[18] Many of these methods are used for practicing interactions with clients in either small or large animal settings.[12] The author was unable to determine if institutions were using these types of methods to provide practice interactions with the veterinary team as the setting. As early as 2003, simulated clients have been incorporated into veterinary curriculum.[11] The clients could be students posing as the client or hired actors. In many instances, the interactions are videotaped and then reviewed by the student involved, faculty-in-charge of the class, or small groups of peers.[11] In some instances, having the actor provide feedback is also included.[19] The ability to practice "real life" scenarios for students prior to entering the final year of clinical rotation is invaluable so that they may be better prepared to handle a difficult client, euthanasia discussions, or quality of life discussions.

However, there are articles regarding some difficulties in implementation. For example, simulated clients tend to be white females according to Soltero and colleagues[20] when they did a survey of institutions that use actors for simulated clients. Without a diversity of clients, students may not learn about their own biases about different groups from themselves and their communication style may not work in those situations. Cultural competence and cultural humility are concepts that need a diversity of simulated clients and educational instruction to improve the practice of veterinary medicine.[21–23]

Some institutions have implemented experiential learning opportunities that have students interact with various communities that perhaps they would normally not engage with. Some examples include WisCARES,[13] a low cost veterinary medical teaching clinic working with low income or unhoused pet owners, University of Florida's Pets are Wonderful Support (PAWS) program[15] working with disabled low income clients and in Canada, working with indigenous communities[14] via the University of Calgary. The students in these experiences overall liked the experiences and allowed them to gain practical experiences in communicating with clients different from themselves. Adding to the diversity of simulated clients, for example, a physical disability, body shape, gender identity, language differences, and socioeconomic status, can be a way to include DEI into communications without having it centered on race or ethnicity as the only DEI topics to know.

EXTRACURRICULAR PROGRAMMING AND EVENTS

Student clubs are a valuable source of programming and learning opportunities for the professional students outside the classroom and there are many different types from student chapters of national organizations like the American Association of Bovine Practitioners, American Society of Laboratory Animal Medicine, and Shelter Medicine or Zoo Medicine to just name a few. There are also veterinary fraternities that students can join for social activities. Many of these clubs invite speakers or offer experiential learning opportunities for students throughout the year to gain exposure to various aspects of the veterinary profession. Opportunity for belonging for historically marginalized students can be improved by inviting different speakers versus the same ones every year. For example, inviting a female large animal practitioner instead of a male practitioner can help those women identifying students see that it is possible.[24] This is where some of the student affinity groups come in by inviting speakers of various fields in veterinary medicine to speak about how they were able to get into their field or specialty. With the capability of videoconferencing improving due to the coronavirus disease 2019 pandemic, inviting speakers from different states or even countries to participate in panels is possible. By seeing people who look like you doing what you want to do professionally, it makes it more possible to do for students and increase the feeling of belonging.[4,5,25] This sense of belonging has improved success rates of completion at the undergraduate education level.[25] This can be extended to veterinary students or other health professional students.[26,27] Experiential learning can be a requirement for some clubs. For example, VOICE has an outreach component in order to receive funding from the national sponsor according to the bylaws.[28] These activities provide a 2-fold opportunity. Students gaining experience under the guidance of a faculty advisor for pet health clinics, after school programs, and so forth and the public sees the veterinary students from various backgrounds doing the work, serving as a role model to younger children or students. NABV also has an outreach component requirement to have a student chapter. The chapter can do outreach to undergraduate students and or high school students.[29]

Faculty can also contribute to the feeling of belonging or lack thereof. The article by Kramper and colleagues[30] demonstrated how students who identify as part of the LGBTQIA + community experienced discrimination or harassment not only from classmates, but also from faculty, supervisors, and clients. When asked how it was resolved, 27% indicated that it was not resolved while 14.5% indicated that they found another place of employment or graduated. Similar experiences occur for racial or ethnic minority students with faculty mistaking marginalized students for each other on rotations or in class.[4] While many faculties do not make these mistakes, few do anything to correct the situation if it occurs in front of them. Kessler and Varnado published a paper discussing how white faculty can be allies in the classroom.[31] Here, they suggest the JEDI Code where JEDI stands for justice, equity, diversity and inclusion, be implemented in the classroom. They discuss how to provide a structure and culture for the classroom where all students can be successful, regardless of background. This includes expectations of student behavior, equity practices by the faculty member in class, reflective facilitation time, and other universal teaching design elements. However, the changing landscape of DEI being taught in the classroom may cause some professional programs to figure new ways that do not run against state legislation or state mandates. Most of these laws have been aimed at the K-12 education levels but several now are taking aim at college level education, which may impact accreditation.[8] One state governor has even sued the federal government regarding accreditation.[32,33] Part of the COE accreditation of veterinary schools is that the hosting university is accredited by an authorized governing body.[1]

Programming by non-university entities can also help with creating a belonging and inclusive culture and provide educational opportunities for faculty and staff to learn along with students. AAVMC hosts several podcasts a year with its Diversity on Air podcast (hosted by Dr Lisa Greenhill) that people can watch live or view later on a variety of DEI topics. Dr Greenhill also hosts various book club reads on topics of diversity that are not strictly veterinary related. The AAVMC annual meeting that is aimed at veterinary administrators, faculty and staff has a DEI track as part of its educational program. The AVMA has also started offering more DEI Continuing Education (CE) credits at its annual meeting in the professional development track. The other major continuing education meetings are also including DEI programming with CE credit as ways for practicing veterinary professionals to learn more. Even some of the veterinary specialty boards now have non-medical CE credit lectures and webinars that focus on DEI topics. As an example, The Davis-Thompson Foundation hosted “Voices in Pathology”, a webinar series, which focused on race or ethnicity and gender or sexual orientation of its members and their struggles to overcome obstacles based on those identities. Some state veterinary medical associations are also hosting non-medical CE credit workshops and webinars for their members on a variety of DEI topics.

CLINICS CARE POINTS

- Communication and cultural humility are critical skills when interacting with clients.
- Groups during veterinary school and as a professional provide feelings of belonging.

DISCLOSURE

The author has no conflicts of interest.

REFERENCES

1. Accreditation Policies and Procedures of the AVMA Council on Education (COE), Secondary accreditation policies and procedures of the AVMA Council on Education (COE), Available at: https://www.avma.org/education/center-for-veterinary-accreditation/accreditation-policies-and-procedures-avma-council-education-coe, (Accessed February 7, 2024). 2024.

2. Molgaard LK, Hodgson JL, Bok HGJ, et al. Competecy-based veterinary education part 1: CBVE framework. In: . Washington, DC: Association of American Veterinary Medical Colleges; 2018.
3. Cheng SM, Taylor DL, Fitzgerald AA, et al. Build & belong: a peer-based intervention to reduce medical student social isolation. Teach Learn Med 2022;34(5): 504–13.
4. Chung CH, Armitage-Chan E. Students experiences and ethnic diversity: the experiences of underrepresented minority students at a Veterinary University in the United Kingdom. J Vet Med Educ 2022;49(3):363–71.
5. Brannon TN, Lin A. "Pride and prejudice" pathways to belonging: implications for inclusive diversity practices within mainstream institutions. Am Psychol 2021; 76(3):488–501.
6. Petersen KH, Jain NR, Case B, et al. Impact of USMLE Step-1 accommodation denial on US medical schools: a national survey. PLoS One 2022;17(4):e0266685.
7. Johnson AD. A review of exam accommodations for dental students with disabilities. J Dent Educ 2006;70(5):475–9.
8. DEI Legislation Tracker. Secondary DEI legislation tracker, Available at: https://www.chronicle.com/article/here-are-the-states-where-lawmakers-are-seeking-to-ban-colleges-dei-efforts, (Accessed February 6, 2024), 2024.
9. Students for Fair admissions, Inc v. President and Fellows of Harvard College; 2023.
10. Students for Fair admissions, Inc v. University of North Carolina; 2023.
11. Radford AD, Stockley P, Taylor IR, et al. Use of simulated clients in training veterinary undergraduates in communication skills. Vet Rec 2003;152(14):422–7.
12. McDermott MP, Tischler VA, Cobb MA, et al. Veterinarian-client communication skills: current state, relevance, and opportunities for improvement. J Vet Med Educ 2015;42(4):305–14.
13. Alvarez E, Lygo-Baker S, Schultz K, et al. Veterinary and pharmacy students' expectations before and experiences after partcipating in an interdisciplinary access to care veterinary clinic. WisCARES. J Vet Med Educ 2022;49(5):610–7.
14. Tsimaras T, Wallace JE, Adams C, et al. Actualizing cultural humility: an exploratory study of veterinary students' participation in a northern community health rotation. J Vet Med Educ 2023;50(2):205–16.
15. Otero DK, James TG, Stone AE. Evaluation of a student-led community-based veterinary clinic for disabled low-income clients: a case study of the university of florida PAWS program. J Vet Med Educ 2023;e20230032.
16. Hammond S, Runion K. Deveopment of a 1-week intensive course on diversity and equity in veterinary medicine. J Vet Med Educ 2022;49(1):8–15.
17. Byrnes MK. Professional skills teaching within veterinary education and possible future directions. J Vet Med Educ 2022;49(6):686–92.
18. Kurtz S. Teaching and learning communication in veterinary medicine. J Vet Med Educ 2006;33(1):11–9.
19. Rauch M, Bettermann V, Tipold A, et al. Use of actors or peers as simulated clients in veterinary communication training. J Vet Med Educ 2023;50(3):314–26.
20. Soltero E, Villalobos CD, Englar RE, et al. Evaluating communication training at AVMA COE-Accredited Institutions and the need to consider diversity within simulated client pools. J Vet Med Educ 2023;50(2):192–204.
21. Gongora J, van Gelderen I, Vost M, et al. Cultural competence is everyone's business: embedding cultural competence in curriculum frameworks to advance veterinary education. J Vet Med Educ 2023;50(1):1–14.

22. Alvarez EE, Gilles WK, Lygo-Baker S, et al. Teaching cultural humility and implicit bias to veterinary medical students: a review and recommendation for best practices. J Vet Med Educ 2020;47(1):2–7.
23. Alvarez EE, Gilles WK, Lygo-Baker S, et al. How to approach cultural humility debriefing within clinical veterinary environments. J Vet Med Educ 2021;48(3): 256–62.
24. Morello SL, Rogus-Pulia N, Branchaw JL, et al. The influence of messaging on perceptions of careers in veterinary medicine: do gender stereotypes matter? J Vet Med Educ 2022;49(3):382–92.
25. Stryhorn TL. College students' sense of belonging: a key to educational success for all students. 2nd edition. New York: Routledge; 2018.
26. Knox-Kazimierczak FA, Tosolt B, Lotz KV. Cultivating a sense of belonging in allied health education: an approach based on mindfulness anti-oppression pedagogy. Health Promot Pract 2023. https://doi.org/10.1177/15248399231172761.
27. Greenhill LM, Davis KC, Lowrie PM, Amass SF. editors.Navigating diversity and inclusion in veterinary medicine. Lafayette (IN: Purdue University Press; West; 2013.
28. VOICE, Secondary VOICE, Available at: https://vetvoicenational.wordpress.com/. (Accessed February 16 2024).
29. National Association of Black Veterinarians, Secondary national association of black veterinarians, Available at: https://nabvonline.org/. (Accessed February 16, 2024).
30. Kramper S, Brydon C, Carmichael KP, et al. "The Damage Happens....You Just Try Not to Dwell on It": experiences of discrimination by gender sexual minority veterinary professional and students in the US and the UK. J Vet Med Educ 2023;50(4):482–96.
31. Kessler A, Varnado K. White faculty as true allies in the classroom: the JEDI code. J Allied Health 2022;51(4):292–6.
32. Beltan N. DeSantis challenges federal college accreitation rules. Indep Fla Alligator 2023.
33. Knott K. DeSantis challenges constitutionality of accreditation. Inside Higher Ed; 2023.

Recruiting and Retaining a Diverse Veterinary Team

Charles D. McMillan, DVM

KEYWORDS

• Diversity and inclusion • Hiring • Recruiting • Work culture • Retention

KEY POINTS

- Diversity hiring initiatives require intentionality and mechanisms placed to track and monitor what is and is not working.
- Diverse teams outperform nondiverse teams and deliver higher financial outcomes.
- An inclusive workplace is paramount to fully benefit from diversity. Without inclusion, we cannot learn from the diverse backgrounds in our work environment.
- Diverse leadership in an organization is essential for sustaining successful recruitment and retention of diverse team members.
- Choosing between talent and diversity is a fallacy. Set measurable criteria for all candidates, then choose those from your qualified pool of applicants who get you closer to your diversity goals.

INTRODUCTION

A few years ago, I was in Atlantic City speaking at a popular veterinary conference when 2 veterinarians, a husband and wife, approached me to ask some questions. I had noticed them at one of my earlier, more widely attended lectures on vaccines. I was pleasantly surprised when I saw them walk in for my final presentation on diversity. Usually, attendance and attention begin to wane by the end of long conferences, but here they were in the front row taking intense notes, hanging on every word, and carefully examining every slide, just as they had for my first lecture.

The couple were practice owners in the rural Midwest, and they were interested in finding more diverse talent. They told me that, aside from a few veterinary assistants or customer service representatives, they had a hard time attracting diverse applicants.

I remember thinking that these 2 had a good chance of successfully diversifying their veterinary team, because they had taken the hard, but crucial first steps in identifying an issue and then seeking advice.

GoodVets West Buckhead, 2275 Marietta Boulevard Northwest, Suite 330, Atlanta, GA 30318, USA
E-mail address: Dr.McMillan@goodVets.com

Vet Clin Small Anim 54 (2024) 785–795
https://doi.org/10.1016/j.cvsm.2024.06.003 **vetsmall.theclinics.com**
0195-5616/24/

Some of what I told them up at that podium will be covered in this article, but in much greater detail. I gave them my email and encouraged them to reach out so I could give them a fuller understanding of the dynamics of recruiting and retaining a diverse veterinary team and coach them along their journey. Unfortunately, I never heard from them, but I hope they were able to meet and maintain their diversity goals. I hope that when they inevitably encountered obstacles, they stayed the course. I hope they were steadfast in their conviction and did not waver in their belief in the power of a diverse workforce.

Recruiting and retaining a diverse veterinary team is a multifaceted, dynamic process that takes intentionality and a resolve that few individuals, let alone companies, care to incorporate.

Despite good research from McKinsey and Company and many others who support the fantastic power of a diverse workforce, skepticism remains, if not on the idea of a diverse workforce, then the process of establishing one. But once we understand that diversity hiring is more about individuals and interactions than processes and tools, we can begin to appeal to the better angels of our nature.

Hiring and maintaining a diverse workforce is a cumulative process that must evolve to stand the test of time and respond to changes in your team, work environment, and outside factors. It is both a reactive and proactive process. It involves learning, unlearning, and often initiating practices and policies that can overcome our collective biases. It requires cultural elasticity and an environment that exudes safety—an environment of rewarded vulnerability.

Diverse hiring and retention efforts often fall short for 2 separate but related reasons: lack of deliberate recruiting efforts and failure to modify the environment that diverse employees are asked to thrive in.

Much of what is covered in this article is multidisciplinary and applicable across many fields. It is the author's belief that the best practical application for this article is as a reference, to visit relevant sections as circumstances arise in your journey to a more diverse veterinary team.

BENEFITS OF A DIVERSE WORKFORCE

American worldwide consulting firm McKinsey and Company has conducted studies evaluating the link between diversity and company financial performances.[1] They found that companies with high racial and ethnic diversity among their employees outperformed their counterparts by 35%. Additionally, they found that more diverse companies enjoy 2.3 times higher cash flow per employee.

According to research by Boston Consulting Group,[2] companies that reported above-average diversity on their management teams also reported innovation revenue 19 percentage points higher than companies with below-average leadership diversity.

In a white paper titled "Hacking Diversity with Inclusive Decision-Making," research from Cloverpop[3] found that more diverse teams made better business decisions 87% of the time compared to individual decision-makers, leading to better business performance.

But beyond the numbers, it is important to understand how and why diverse teams excel. This understanding is paramount to functional team building and developing environments that cultivate success. The key is not to simply hire a mix of individuals, but to truly value and learn from their differences. This diversity enriches the organization, fosters innovation, and strengthens the team. To work properly, there must be a commitment to inclusion: that is, respecting and leveraging the differences that diverse voices offer. Diversity without inclusion undermines team success and further marginalizes those from diverse backgrounds.

When diverse teams interact, a cross-pollination occurs that unlocks innovation and stimulates new thinking. This gives them access to unique, complex solutions that might not be obtained by less diverse teams.

Notably, there are 2 types of diversity: inherent and acquired. Inherent diversity involves traits you are born with, such as gender, ethnicity, and sexual orientation. Acquired diversity involves traits you gain from experience. To be successful and maximize potential, organizations and institutions should maximize both. You can never have too much diversity, and these types are not mutually exclusive.

Besides positive financial implications and greater innovation, diverse teams have greater customer understanding. This makes sense, because the world we live in is incredibly diverse and our customer base largely reflects this. Through better customer understanding comes greater access to care, which is vital in the field of veterinary medicine.

During the coronavirus disease 2019 pandemic, there was an information chasm with certain communities on the margins. Mistrust bred skepticism and ultimately led to a breach in access to care. Unsurprisingly, the communities that needed information the most suffered the worst outcomes.

Because of this, pandemic experts implored local leaders, clergyman, and prominent figures in these communities to speak out and engage their neighbors so that the knowledge was received and processed. The thought behind this is that people tend to trust information from those who look and sound like them and/or come from similar backgrounds.

According to the Bureau of Labor Statistics, veterinary medicine is one of the United States' least diverse fields. Juxtapose this with how diverse pet owners are, and we begin to understand a key component of the access to care crisis. There is no more existential threat to access to care than a homogeneous industry attempting to serve a sundry population.

Access to care can be broken down into 5 components: accessibility, affordability, availability, accommodation, and acceptability. I want to focus on acceptability, or how comfortable the client is with the more immutable characteristics of the provider, and vice versa. These characteristics include the age, sex, social status, and ethnicity of provider and client, as well as the client's diagnosis and type of coverage.[4] In short, clients and customers are more likely to go and (more importantly) keep going to places where the environment makes them feel comfortable. Some of the things that make clients feel comfortable are having service/care providers who look and sound like them and who are from similar walks of life. More pertinently, a team with a member who shares a client's ethnicity is 152% likelier than another team to understand that client.[5]

Customers want to feel heard no matter what background they come from, but for those from historically devalued intersectional identities, the emphasis is even greater.

Having a diverse veterinary team is a dynamic business strategy that can spark innovation, enhance customer relationships, and drive business growth. It also raises your hospital or business's reputation, thereby attracting more talented employees. Conceptually, people have little trouble understanding the inherent benefits of diversity—especially we in the medical profession—whether that means the biodiversity in fruitful ecosystems, diversity in our genetic makeup, pollination and seed dispersal, or climate regulation. But understanding and unlocking the power of diversity is one thing. It is quite another to attract, recruit, and retain a diverse workforce.

STRATEGIES FOR RECRUITING AND HIRING A DIVERSE VETERINARY TEAM

There are many ways for a recruiting apparatus to become successful, but it must be 2 things: intentional and goal-oriented. There are certainly other approaches, but without these 2 pillar concepts, recruiting for a more diverse team will be ineffective. Successful recruiting must be active instead of passive, which often, in this scenario, means going where your target employees are. Fancy slogans and "equal opportunity" statements on your hiring page are not enough. You need to actively seek these candidates, and in certain circumstances, you need to create a mechanism that eliminates existing barriers to their application. Intentionality and a goal-oriented mindset will switch the impetus from "We welcome or encourage all interested parties to apply" to aggressively sourcing candidates, developing them, and leveling the playing field as they matriculate through the interview process. Intentional, goal-oriented recruiting requires establishing a pipeline that, if well maintained, will act as your company's wellspring for years to come.

Create Inclusive Job Descriptions

You want to make sure your job descriptions are well thought out, contain deliberate messaging, clearly state your companies' goals and values, and do not come off as performative, which could deter certain candidates.

Diversity initiatives should involve more than rainbow-faced photos on your career landing page, and whenever possible, you should use pictures of your actual employees. (If you have no diverse employees to include in ads, that should be impetus enough to get the ball rolling.) Recruiting initiatives should reach groups where they are comfortable and spend the most time. Using advanced marketing technology, you can specifically target certain demographics and raise your companies' social profile within certain groups.

In a Harvard Business Review article titled "Stop Making the Business Case for Diversity," the authors conclude that companies making the business case for why they value diversity in their job ads has negative effects on diverse candidates.

> *Most organizations don't feel the need to explain why they care about core values such as innovation, resilience, or integrity. And yet when it comes to diversity, lengthy justifications of the value of hiring a diverse workforce have become the norm in corporate America and beyond.*

Underrepresented job seekers were relatively more receptive to companies making a "fairness" case for diversity over a business case, but not by much. Participants "who read a business case for diversity on average anticipated feeling 11% less sense of belonging to the company, were 16% more concerned that they would be stereotyped at the company and were 10% more concerned that the company would view them as interchangeable with other members of their identity group, compared to those who read a fairness case," the article goes on to say. But making a moral or fairness case for diversity hiring was also met with trepidations from minority job seekers. One of the authors summarized, "The issue with the fairness case is, I contend, it risked tokenizing diverse coworkers, because instead of them having an ostensible value add to the company, their presence might have been just viewed as—having them here is the right/'fair' thing to do."

The authors conclude that best practice is to include neither a business nor fairness case for diversity. Instead, they suggest that, as with any other core value, no justification is needed.

I, however, reject this notion. I would agree if diversity was like any other core value. Not mentioning why you think it is important that your company be as diverse as possible is a cop-out and lets companies off the hook. Furthermore, the issue is framed incorrectly by saying, "Most organizations don't feel the need to explain why they care about core values such as innovation, resilience, or integrity," because the benefits of those core values are more inherently known to the general public. It is reasonable to assume that some people might be unaware of the benefits companies gain through diversity. This is especially salient in hyperhomogenous companies, where the inclination might be that upholding the status quo is just fine.

My preference would be that companies explain all their core values as opposed to not explaining any. This dialogic process must also include current employees, as they can be your best evangelists, especially if they are aware of what your company is doing to increase diversity.

In the end, job descriptions should be deliberate. They should include your goals and the reasoning behind your core values. They should also be discussed with your team first to get buy-in and so your employees can vouch for the work your company is doing behind the scenes to hire and retain diverse members.

Expanding Your Hiring Pool

When you are looking to add something that has been eluding your company, you need to go where that missing thing is: "fish where the fish are." This could mean reaching out to diverse job boards, professional groups, or historically Black colleges and universities. Partnering with organizations that advocate for underrepresented groups can also connect you with more diverse candidates. These connections should foster a relationship that educates future candidates about the opportunities you have available and why they should consider working for your company. Your interactions should not only encourage qualified applicants to apply but also eliminate any barriers to applying. Detailed record keeping is imperative so you can track the responsiveness to your different outreach efforts. If there is interest from candidates who do not immediately qualify, this outreach should also include clear steps on how they can become qualified, and have tracking mechanisms to monitor their progress.

Embrace Unbiased Hiring

We are unlikely to ever reach a place where biases stop developing, as most biases start at an early age and occur at the subconscious level. The goal with unbiased hiring is to create systems that prevent biases from resulting in discrimination. Biases permeate the entire hiring apparatus, and there must be practices and policies in place to mitigate their deleterious effects.

Sociologist Devah Pager performed a hiring study[6] in Milwaukee, Wisconsin, comparing the likelihoods of receiving job callbacks between 2 comparable groups only distinguished by race. A group of Black applicants and a group of White applicants applied for the same job. The job required no experience and only a high school education. The study concluded that White applicants were twice as likely as equally qualified Black applicants to receive a callback. To accentuate the point, White applicants who listed a criminal record on their resumes received more callbacks than did comparable Black applicants without a criminal record.

In another notable investigation, economists Marianne Bertrand and Sendhil Mullainathan explored hiring practices by deploying a vast array of fabricated resumes in response to job postings across Chicago and Boston newspapers.[7] These resumes, tailored for various positions, were nearly identical except for the names, with half featuring African American-sounding names and the other half bearing names typically associated with White individuals. Subsequent tracking of callback rates revealed stark disparities: resumes with White-sounding names garnered 50% more interview invitations. The researchers summarized their findings by stating that while a White applicant might reasonably anticipate one callback for every 10 applications, an

African American applicant would need to submit around 15 applications to achieve comparable results.

As the earlier studies show, minority candidates experience increasing difficulty in reaching the interview process. Once there, affinity biases and in-group favoritism are 2 of many factors that can prevent qualified applicants from underrepresented backgrounds from getting the job.

One possible way to circumvent biases during the hiring process is by blinding applicant resumes, that is, by removing indications of gender, ethnicity, and sexual orientation. Stated differently, it involves blocking evaluators from receiving potentially biasing information about a job candidate until after evaluation of their application materials is complete.

Some diverse candidates, frustrated with facing inequities, have resorted to "whitening" their resumes. This involves removing mentions of memberships and positions in obviously African American organizations and altering or omitting names of traditionally Black colleges or universities.

But eventually there will be an interview, and candidates cannot hide their race, gender, and ethnicity forever. How, then, do we protect these candidates during the interview process?

Foster Diversity from the Top Down

If intentionality stirs your diversity recruiting program, then diverse leadership provides the critical wind behind the sails. Companies must have not only leadership that is committed to diversity but also diverse leaders. When leadership can be seen participating in diversity and inclusion efforts, this sends a substantial message to the rest of the organization and sets its tone.

The influence of social norms underscores the importance of collective attitudes toward diversity within an organization. When everyone else in the company appears to prioritize diversity, individuals are more inclined to align their behavior accordingly. Conversely, if attitudes toward diversity are indifferent or instances of prejudice and discrimination are tolerated, they can become ingrained as norms, undermining diversity efforts and reducing them to mere symbolic gestures.

You should notice a theme throughout the article: diverse leadership is a vital cog in both recruiting and retention of a diverse team, an informative and aspirational marker to potential candidates and current employees alike.

Recruiting and retaining a diverse veterinary team is less about hiring individuals from different backgrounds, and more about fostering an environment where everyone has equal opportunities to succeed.

Having diversity in leadership positions transcends simple representation: it adds representation in places where policies and decisions are made. Without it, support that minorities receive can be inadequate, as people (including leaders) tend to be favorably biased toward others who share similar backgrounds or remind them of themselves. Without diverse leadership, women are 20% less likely than straight White men to win endorsement for their ideas; people of color are 24% less likely; and lesbian, gay, bisexual, and transgender (LGBT) people are 21% less likely.[5]

Having diverse leadership disrupts this dogma, leading toward more equitable opportunities for advancements within an organization.

Be Goal-oriented, Not Process-oriented

The essence of every recruiting apparatus is the approach we choose to achieve the outcomes we desire. There have been many celebrated rules and policies enacted at the highest levels of business to address hiring disparities. Some have been successful, while others have failed or undergone permutations after retrospective data showed a degree of ineffectiveness.

One of the most famous approaches to diversity hiring is the Rooney rule of the National Football League (NFL). The rule mandated that NFL teams interview at least one minority candidate for every head coaching opening. The NFL adopted it in response to legal threats over the massive disparity between the number of Black head coaches in relation to the number of Black players. In a league where roughly 70% of players are Black, the anemic numbers of Black head coaches had long needed to be addressed.

While the Rooney rule initially seemed to work and was met with praise and the highest form of flattery—adoption by other organizations—years later, the NFL reverted back to form.

Diverse candidates, eager for opportunity, initially welcomed such rules, as they provided much-needed exposure. Interviews were a chance to showcase their capabilities to potential employers. However, the rule's implementation across other organizations became rife with misbehavior, workarounds, fake interviews, and fake results, eventually acting as a tool to tokenize and further relegate diverse candidates.

The Mansfield Rule, implemented by numerous major law firms in 2017, mandates that at least 30% of candidates considered for high-level positions must be people of color, women, or individuals from other underrepresented groups. While credited with enhancing diversity within firms, this rule has faced criticism. Paola Cecchi DiMeglio, a data scientist at Harvard Law School, contends that the rule "has had no effect," attributing improved numbers to shifting national demographics.

The failure of the Rooney Rule is largely attributed to NFL owners' lack of seriousness toward its implementation and the absence of significant institutional oversight or league sanctions against those circumventing its intent. Attorney Linda Friedman, who has filed racial discrimination lawsuits against major financial firms, said, "It's not the idea that failed—it's the rollout." She added, "If you're going to introduce it to an institution uninterested in change, it won't matter what you introduce. It won't stick."

Whether an organization has adopted a rule like those outlined earlier or has decided to expend energy and resources on seeking equality in other ways, their initiatives can be grouped into 2 categories: process-oriented and goal-oriented.

Process-oriented programs focus on creating a fair application process, assuming that this will result in a fair outcome. The issue with some process-oriented programs is that bias can affect applicant selection very early in the search.

Goal-oriented approaches address some of the limitations of process-oriented methods by continually evaluating the diversity of the candidate pool at each stage of hiring. This involves investigating whether the pool is sufficiently diverse and whether efforts have been made to attract a broad range of applicants. In a goal-oriented approach, candidates who advance the company's diversity objectives are prioritized from among the qualified pool. While this does not guarantee that underrepresented candidates will always be selected, it can increase the likelihood that candidates from diverse backgrounds will succeed.

RETAINING YOUR DIVERSE WORKFORCE

So far, we have discussed processes and techniques to attract and hire a diverse veterinary team, as well as the thinking behind them. Equally important, if not more so, is how to retain the diverse group of talent you have acquired.

Assimilation versus Inclusion

Diversity does not work without inclusion. In fact, without inclusion, diversity numbers will flatten, and initiatives aimed at increasing diversity will have the opposite effect. When you juxtapose the word "diversity" with "inclusion," it suggests a distinction between concepts; however, the 2 words can be viewed as different ways to approach diversity management. To activate the power of diverse voices, these voices must feel welcomed and appreciated for what they have to offer. Furthermore, inclusion goes beyond invitation to involve actively seeking participation from all groups. This participation should be taken seriously, and individuals should be rewarded and acknowledged for their thoughtful contributions.

Assimilation stands in opposition to inclusion. Here, it involves adopting the cultural norms of a dominant group, often placing the burden on marginalized individuals. They are pressured to conform, avoiding any disruption to the majority's comfort. Jacobs and colleagues in their Harvard Business Review article "Do Your Diversity Initiatives Promote Assimilation over Inclusion?" assert that not having to invest social and mental energy into assimilation is a privilege. They further highlight that this demand for conformity exacts emotional and mental tolls, hindering personal and professional development.[8] The key here is creating an environment where your diverse employees are emboldened to contribute something to your work culture instead of assimilating into it.

Psychological Safety

The feeling that enables people to freely speak out and contribute is called psychological safety. It is an environment of rewarded vulnerability. To maximize the unique gifts of any diverse work team, you must have psychological safety.

Intuitively, we can see how psychological safety is imperative. In his article "Agile Doesn't Work Without Psychological Safety," author Timothy R. Clark puts its succinctly, saying, "High psychological safety elicits a performance response with innovation as the goal, whereas low psychological safety elicits a fear response with survival as the goal."[9]

Peer/Affinity Groups

You can offer support to your diversity initiatives by facilitating groups that connect employees with others of similar identities and backgrounds. These are often called employee resource groups or affinity groups. If your individual hospital or clinic does not have a large enough population of diverse employees yet, you can provide information on external groups, or start one by pooling resources with neighboring hospitals or hospital groups.

Participants may find group meetings beneficial to connect with a variety of colleagues and seek advice on coping with certain situations. While these meetings may not occur daily, "they are important for psychological survival in such situations," writes Dr Beverly Daniel Tatum in her seminal book *Why Are All the Black Kids Sitting Together in the Cafeteria?*

Developing or taking advantage of these groups is most important in the neonatal stages of building a diverse workforce, because until numbers grow, members of underrepresented groups may feel tokenized and isolated and "joining with one's peers for support in the face of stress is a positive coping strategy," Dr Tatum writes.[10]

Having diverse leadership to help spearhead and even participate in these group settings helps marginalized employees feel heard and enables access to powerful leadership structures. This, in turn, facilitates these employees becoming embedded in networks that might not otherwise be available to them. Getting senior executives from all backgrounds involved will also support recruiting, retention, and heightened employee productivity.

Thoughtful Feedback Modules

Feedback is particularly important for your diverse team members in leadership roles. In a Harvard Business Review article titled "Research: Men Get More Actionable Feedback Than Women," the authors state that "managers are more likely to give actionable and in-the-moment feedback to men than women. Similar dynamics have been observed based on race, ability, and sexual orientation."[11]

Intuitively, it is easy to imagine that employees who are not given usable feedback start to flounder in the workplace and eventually become frustrated at a lack of career advancement. Further, lack of actionable feedback can be a demotivator and lead to high attrition rates.

In the same Harvard Business Review article, the authors write, "At most organizations, there is less diversity at higher levels. As more women and people of color achieve higher levels of leadership, there is more pressure to be successful, set an example for others, and 'justify' their role." This creates a disengagement loop, as diverse leaders may become reluctant to seek feedback for fear of being perceived as weak leaders or "less than." By extension, this impedes organizational growth and can precipitate workplace failure. The shortcomings of one diverse leader tend to reverberate in the minds of the majority group, causing a reluctance by those in power to give another leadership opportunity to a member of a diverse group due to the "out-group homogeneity effect."

Frequent, useful feedback should be given to all employees at all levels in order for them to stay engaged and productive for your company.

Fair and Competitive Compensation

Having selected an underrepresented candidate from a qualified pool of applicants by applying what you have learned from the recruiting section, you should offer a salary that is commensurate with their skills and in line with your company's equitable compensation guidelines for that position. Pay should be based on merit regardless of race, gender, or ethnicity.

Despite this sentiment, pay gaps persist and have a compounding effect on ethnically diverse candidates, as they, according to the American Association of Veterinary Medical Colleges (AAVMC), graduate with higher student loan debt after veterinary school.[12] While not en vogue for many industries, particularly veterinary medicine, salary transparency is a path to better job satisfaction.

CONTROVERSY AROUND HIRING FOR DIVERSITY

The main argument against diversity initiatives is that they contravene meritocracy. Some people believe that meritocracy and diversity are incompatible. In a meritocracy, societal advancements occur based on an individual's capabilities and merits rather than their family, wealth, or social background.

Organizations that reject diversity initiatives do so believing that their companies are meritocratic. They argue that if a woman or person of color is qualified, they will be hired and promoted. Diversity initiatives, therefore, are unnecessary and could potentially compromise quality. The essence of the argument is 2 fold: (1) hiring for diversity necessarily sacrifices quality and (2) everyone who is qualified and wants a job has equal access to it.

Belief in a true meritocracy aligns with the notion of a "just world," as described by Dr Tatum, author of *Why Are All the Black Kids Sitting Together in the Cafeteria?* It suggests that individuals receive what they deserve based on their actions and efforts. However, this belief overlooks the reality of unfair advantages and differing starting points, particularly affecting marginalized groups, especially those with multiple intersecting identities. Psychologist John Dovidio terms this denial of effects as color-blind ideology, where White individuals minimize or deny racial inequality, attributing contemporary disparities to factors unrelated to race.[13]

Organizations with homogenous workforces invalidate the idea of operating as a meritocracy, not the other way around. Furthermore, if organizations are prioritizing merit and certain sociodemographic groups are still underrepresented, then that suggests either a lack of interest or aptitude inherent in the underrepresented groups. This becomes a biological deterministic argument, suggesting inferior characteristics within a group that make them unsuitable for appointment to a certain role.

SUMMARY

As our country becomes increasingly diverse, our workforces must reflect this change to remain acceptable in the eyes of our consumers and serve more of the population. While recruiting and retaining a diverse veterinary team may seem more challenging in some geographic sectors, it is important that we enact intentional processes that will afford our workforces the greatest chance of obtaining the rich diversity our industry desperately needs.

We have touched on the myriad benefits of a diverse team, but less obvious, and perhaps more damaging, are the insidious effects on our industry should we fail to achieve a more inclusive future.

After assembling your diverse veterinary team, meticulously scouring your work environment to uproot any impediments to retaining them is essential if you are to unlock their benefits.

Diversity and talent should never be made to stand in opposition. They go together like needle and yarn, knitting the fabric of our collected humanity.

When we look around at our team meetings, board rooms, and executive retreats, there should be an assortment of people from different backgrounds. If you frequently find that this is not the case, pick up this article and let us begin this journey together.

DISCLOSURE

The author has nothing to disclose.

REFERENCES

1. McKinsey and Company. Delivering through diversity. 2018. Available at: https://www.mckinsey.com/capabilities/people-and-organizational-performance/our-insights/delivering-through-diversity. [Accessed 24 March 2024].
2. Boston Consulting Group (BCG). How diverse leadership teams boost innovation. 2018. Available at: https://www.bcg.com/publications/2018/how-diverse-leadership-teams-boost-innovation. [Accessed 24 March 2024].
3. Cloverpop. Hacking diversity with inclusive decision-making. Publication date not provided. Available at: https://www.cloverpop.com/hubfs/Whitepapers/Cloverpop_Hacking_Diversity_Inclusive_Decision_Making_White_Paper.pdf. [Accessed 24 March 2024].

4. McLaughlin CG, Wyszewianski L. Access to care: remembering old lessons. Health Serv Res 2002 Dec;37(6):1441–3.
5. Hunt V, Prince S, Dixon-Fyle S, et al. How diversity can drive innovation. Harv Bus Rev 2018. Available at: https://hbr.org/2018/12/how-diversity-can-drive-innovation.
6. Pager D. The Mark of a Criminal Record. 2003.
7. Bertrand M, Mullainathan S. Are Emily and Greg more employable than Lakisha and Jamal? A field experiment on labor market discrimination. NBER Working Paper Series. Working Paper 9873; 2003. Available at: http://www.nber.org/papers/w9873.
8. Carey L. Do your diversity initiatives promote assimilation over inclusion? Harv Bus Rev 2019. Available at: https://hbr.org/2019/06/do-your-diversity-initiatives-promote-assimilation-over-inclusion.
9. Edmondson A. Agile doesn't work without psychological safety. Harv Bus Rev 2019. Available at: https://hbr.org/2019/05/agile-doesnt-work-without-psychological-safety.
10. Tatum, B. D. (2003). Why Are All the Black Kids Sitting Together in the Cafeteria?: And Other Conversations About Race. Basic Books.
11. Doldor E, Wyatt M, Silvester J. Research: men get more actionable feedback than women. 2021. Available at: https://hbr.org/2021/02/research-men-get-more-actionable-feedback-than-women. [Accessed 21 March 2023].
12. Internal AAVMC Data Reports. Mean Institutionally Reported Indebtedness at U.S. Colleges of Veterinary Medicine. 2021.
13. Banaji MR, Greenwald AG. Blindspot: hidden biases of good people. Delacorte Press; 2016.

The Value of Qualitative Research in Diversity, Equity, and Inclusion

Sohaila Jafarian, DVM, MPH*

KEYWORDS

- Qualitative research • Epistemic violence • Community-based participatory research
- Emancipatory research • Humanizing research • Liberatory research

KEY POINTS

- Qualitative research offers a necessary complement to quantitative methods in veterinary medicine, providing deeper insight into human experiences.
- The article identifies qualitative research as a tool to combat epistemic violence, ensuring research practices avoid perpetuating harm and marginalization.
- It underscores the value of community-based participatory research and other emancipatory methodologies that position community members as coresearchers and active participants.
- Key frameworks such as humanizing and liberatory approaches are advocated for their potential to transform conventional research into a more inclusive and equitable practice.
- The article concludes with a call to integrate these transformative approaches into veterinary research, promoting a paradigm that values diversity, equity, and inclusion.

INTRODUCTION

This article is intended to help those in the veterinary field understand a research methodology that is not commonly utilized in our field, qualitative research. Initially, we define qualitative research and distinguish it from quantitative research, examining the unique strengths and limitations of each method. This discussion sets the stage for a deeper exploration of why qualitative research is vital in veterinary medicine, especially in contexts that demand a nuanced understanding of diverse experiences and perspectives.

We delve into the concept of epistemic violence and discuss how, traditionally, research has perpetuated harm. To counteract this, we introduce and advocate for

Board Member for Multicultural Veterinary Medical Association and Relief Veterinarian for Jafarian Relief Services, LLC, Albuquerque, NM, USA
* P.O. Box 1742, Silverdale, WA 98383.
E-mail address: JafarianDVM@gmail.com

Vet Clin Small Anim 54 (2024) 797–811
https://doi.org/10.1016/j.cvsm.2024.06.004 vetsmall.theclinics.com

utilizing the strengths of qualitative research in conjunction with approaches such as community-based participatory research (CBPR), along with emancipatory, humanizing, and liberatory frameworks. These approaches not only enrich the research process by involving community members as coresearchers but also challenge and transform conventional perspectives on scientific inquiry. This article aims to illustrate how qualitative research can foster a more inclusive, equitable, and empathetic framework for scientific discovery.

WHAT IS QUALITATIVE RESEARCH?

In veterinary medicine, the majority of research conducted, published, used as resources, and taught is quantitative. This research provides information on specific, quantifiable information such as efficacy of a particular treatment, prevalence of a disease, or evaluation of a new surgical technique. Quantitative research is unable to thoroughly investigate nonquantifiable information, such as people's experiences or opinions. Consequently, what information could we be missing, only utilizing one avenue of scientific exploration? How do we identify gaps in the research? Whose voices, experiences, and opinions are we not hearing or valuing? What other tools do we have to understand veterinary medicine, its role, and its impacts?

Qualitative research is a research methodology that aims to understand the "lived experience" of a specific group of people, gathering information, such as peoples' experiences, perceptions, and emotions, and finding themes and patterns within that data. Thus, qualitative data are looking for information that is not easily quantifiable, such as the processes and patterns of human behavior.[1,2] Qualitative research does not typically generate straightforward answers, but produces studies providing narrative accounts, explanations, typologies of phenomena, and conceptual frameworks.[3]

As explained by Miles and colleagues,[4] "qualitative data are a source of well-grounded, rich descriptions of social processes" and that "good qualitative data also lead to serendipitous findings and interrelationships. They help researchers get beyond initial conceptions and generate new understandings." They elaborate on this point explaining that "Words and images, especially organized into vignettes, stories, and evocative visual representations, have a concrete, vivid, and meaningful flavor that often proves far more persuasive to a reader than pages of summary statistics."

SIMILARITIES WITH QUANTITATIVE RESEARCH

Considering that many professionals in veterinary medicine are more familiar with quantitative research methodologies, it is beneficial to start by exploring how qualitative research parallels with quantitative methodology. From there, we can delve more into the distinctions between the 2 approaches. This comparison will pave the way to a holistic understanding of qualitative research, highlighting its significance and its potential as a tool for emancipatory, humanizing, and liberatory research.

Similar to quantitative research, qualitative methodologies also involve key stages such as data condensation, displaying results, and drawing conclusions. In quantitative research, these stages typically include condensing data through calculations like means and standard deviations, displaying results in formats such as correlation tables and regression printouts, and drawing conclusions or verifying hypotheses by examining significance levels and differences between experimental and control groups.[4]

DIFFERENCES WITH QUANTITATIVE RESEARCH

The methodologies of qualitative and quantitative research differ significantly in several key areas, including the formulation of research questions, sample sizes, sampling techniques, and the pursuit of universal applicability in results.

In contrast to quantitative research, where the research question is typically established at the beginning and remains fixed, qualitative research approaches this differently with a more fluid approach. The research question in qualitative studies may be defined at the outset, evolve, or even emerge during the fieldwork; it may also undergo revision and refinement based on emerging data.

Qualitative research generally involves smaller sample sizes than quantitative research, which seeks large numbers to achieve statistical significance. While quantitative studies often utilize random sampling to ensure generalizability, qualitative sampling is usually strategic and purposive, emphasizing the in-depth exploration of specific contexts and phenomena.

Furthermore, quantitative research often employs instruments that abstract data from their contexts to ensure uniformity and comparability across different settings. In contrast, qualitative research is deeply embedded in specific situational contexts, focusing on the particularities that produce generalities, not the other way around.[4]

While the qualitative research methodology may seem antithetical to quantitative research, they cannot be simply categorized as opposites or incompatible.[1,5] Rather, both research methodologies bring different strengths to academic exploration and are often utilized simultaneously in mixed-methods investigations. The most common cited reasons for utilizing a mixed-methods methodology are (1) to add analytical texture to the work, (2) to compensate for the deficiencies of one methodology with the strengths of another, and (3) to modify or strengthen the results of each methodology to support, corroborate, or contradict each other.[4]

STRENGTHS OF QUALITATIVE RESEARCH

One of the major strengths of qualitative research is understanding the lived experience of a specific group. Lived experience is a representation and understanding of a participant's experiences, choices, and options and how those factors influence one's perception of knowledge.[6] Thus, the focus is on naturally occurring, everyday events in their natural settings, so that we can locate the meanings people place on the events, processes, and structures of their lives and connect those meanings to the social world around them. Because the data in qualitative research are typically collected in close proximity to a specific situation, there is a local groundedness, signifying a focused and bounded phenomenon embedded in its context.[4]

Due to the fact that qualitative data collect a large amount of data, frequently over an extended and sustained period, it has a strong potential for "revealing complexity." To quote Miles and colleagues,[4] "We can go far beyond snapshots of 'what?' or 'how many?' to just how and why things happen as they do—and even assess causation as it actually plays out in a particular setting." This depth is crucial in revealing the multilayered nature of human experiences and social interactions.

Transitioning from these foundational strengths, qualitative research excels in rendering the social dimensions of life through evocative prose that transports readers into the field. This immersion is achieved through what Saldaña describes as,[4] "significant trivia"—the detailed, vivid imagery that gives a palpable sense of place and person. This technique not only enhances the narrative but also enriches the reader's understanding of the context.[4]

The flexibility of qualitative methods is evident in that some researchers opt for minimal prestructured designs. Given the complexity and fluidity of social processes, these researchers advocate for a more adaptive, emergent approach. They prioritize inductive reasoning that allows research questions to unfold naturally from the data. This emergent strategy is particularly valuable when exploring new or complex terrains, unfamiliar cultures, understudied phenomena, or very complex social processes, where predefined hypotheses might be limiting.[4]

Correspondingly, qualitative research is not just about exploration and description. It also offers robust tools for hypothesis testing within naturally occurring settings, thereby checking the validity of specific predictions. This capability is crucial when integrating qualitative findings with quantitative data in mixed-methods studies, where qualitative insights can validate, supplement, or illuminate the quantitative aspects, providing a comprehensive view of a research problem.[4]

Qualitative research is also a powerful tool for identifying gaps in research that quantitative research is intrinsically unable to identify, being seen as a strategy for discovery, a methodology for exploring new ideas, and for developing hypotheses.[4] There are numerous interesting and relevant instances of this occurring in the literature.

Take for example, Ryan and colleagues' research on people with long-term conditions,[7] which highlights both a strength of discovery and a weakness of bias in qualitative research. Their secondary analysis utilized data from 6 collections of interviews of carers of people with dementia or multiple sclerosis as well as patient experiences with long-term conditions such as Parkinson's, autism, heart failure, and stroke. The potential that the topic of the place of pets in people's health experiences emerged at an early stage of their secondary analysis, and thus, a broader analysis including any mention of pets was performed. Their study differs from prior research on the role of pets in chronic illness by revisiting interview recordings to investigate complex interactions among participants, pets, and interviewers.

Interestingly, when investigators analyzed the interview recordings, they found that the researchers conducting the interviews had summarized interactions with pets as an unexplained interruption in the transcripts and some researchers had turned off the recording device during those interactions with pets. When reviewing the recordings, investigators discovered that the topic of pets was almost exclusively raised by the participants and not the researchers. Pets were physically excluded from the interview room (by the participant, another member of the household, or the researcher) or labeled as unexplained interruptions in transcripts, suggesting the researchers' disinterest and failure to probe their significance.

Furthermore, it was found that even when the participants presented their pets as important family members, the researchers' reactions to the presence or talk about pets was drastically different than their responses to other household members. Consequently, pets were seldom discussed in the initial analysis and reporting of findings. The authors of the secondary analysis concluded that reconceptualizing the relationship between people and their pets could liberate individuals from self-censorship when discussing this important relationship. This study found that researchers may be contributing to this self-censorship by their inconsistent focus on the role of pets in health. While narrative approaches aim to prioritize participants' interests, they showed clear practical limitations in this study when addressing the significance of pets. While this study illustrates the potential for discovery in qualitative research, it nevertheless demonstrates that even experienced researchers can bring their own biases to a study.

Similarly, in a study of family and kinship, Charles and Davies[8] performed 193 in-depth interviews, and while they did not explicitly ask about animals, a significant portion of their interviewees spontaneously included their pets as part of their kinship networks. Pets were an unanticipated theme and did not become apparent to the researchers until after the interviews were completed. As in the findings by Ryan and colleagues,[7] this study found that the way participants spoke about their pets displayed an uncertainty about how the interviewer may construe that relationship.

A recent qualitative study on veterinary student's experiences on a shelter medicine rotation[9] found that while universities have traditionally focused their shelter medicine educational research on surgical skills gained on rotation with quantitative methodologies, there are more experiences in shelter medicine education that students found deeply fruitful. Students found these unexplored experiences beneficial to their growth as a veterinarian, provided them with takeaways that they found applicable and practical, helped them self-identify significant knowledge gaps, and changed their perspectives on several important topics. Among the conclusions for this study, the researchers concluded that utilizing qualitative research to evaluate student learning experiences needs to be considered to allow for a better understanding of the full context of student learning in academia.

While the strengths of qualitative research are profound in providing rich, contextual insights into complex social phenomena, it is also important to acknowledge its limitations.

WEAKNESSES OF QUALITATIVE RESEARCH

As touched on previously, qualitative research has weak points, just as any research methodology. Qualitative research is inherently more subjective due to its reliance on human experiences and perceptions. This subjectivity can be a double-edged sword: while it allows for rich, detailed insights into complex phenomena, it also opens doors for errors and biases. Researchers' personal characteristics, biases, prejudices, and beliefs can influence every stage of the research process—from conducting interviews and developing codes to the final narrative construction. This influence can skew the research outcomes, leading to conclusions that reflect the researcher's perspective more than the participants'.[10]

The role of the researcher in qualitative studies is significantly more pronounced than in quantitative studies. Their interpretation during interviews, coding practices, and theme development can inadvertently shape the direction and outcomes of the study. The researcher's prior knowledge and biases, either from their personal experiences or cursory review of the literature, can overinfluence interview outlines or affect the choice of themes being formulated, thereby compromising the study's inductive nature.[10]

Grounded theory, a popular analytical approach in qualitative research, faces criticisms regarding the feasibility of conducting a truly inductive analysis free from the researcher's preconceptions. It is nearly impossible to completely set aside one's prior knowledge, which means that every thematic analysis is somewhat influenced by the researcher's previous experiences and theoretic insights. This situation can lead to what is termed "premature theorizing," where themes are shaped by the researcher's expectations rather than purely emerging from the data.[10]

MITIGATING WEAKNESSES

Addressing these weaknesses is crucial for enhancing the validity and relevance of qualitative research and for ensuring that its findings are both robust and reflective of the social phenomena they aim to understand. To address these issues, qualitative researchers employ various strategies. Developing critical subjective awareness is crucial; this involves recognizing and reflecting on the biases that the researcher brings into the process. The concept of "theoretic sensitivity" helps researchers to be explicitly aware of how their existing knowledge influences the research process. Additionally, qualitative research often involves iterative data collection and analysis phases that allow for constant comparison and refinement, helping to ensure that participant perspectives are not overshadowed by the researcher's framework.[10]

By acknowledging and addressing these vulnerabilities, researchers can enhance the rigor of qualitative research and better ensure that findings are both trustworthy and reflective of the studied phenomena.

Numerous studies within the literature have explored methods for assessing quality in qualitative research,[11] team-based qualitative analysis to assess reliability and validity of coded data through intercoder reliability,[12,13] and tactics for researchers to utilize to increase confidence in their findings.[4] However, a detailed exploration of these topics is beyond the scope of this article.

WHY IS QUALITATIVE RESEARCH IMPORTANT?

To appreciate the importance of qualitative research as a tool for understanding peoples' lived experiences, let us begin with an excerpt from *Qualitative Data Analysis: A Methods Sourcebook*.[4]

We believe that social phenomena exist not only in the mind but also in the world—and that some reasonably stable relationships can be found among the idiosyncratic messiness of life. There are regularities and sequences that link together phenomena. From these patterns, we can derive the concepts that underlie individual and social life. The fact that most of those concepts—such as negotiating, possible selves, emotional labor, and so on—are invisible to the human eye does not make them invalid. Human relationships and societies have unique peculiarities and inconsistencies that make a realist approach to understanding them more complex—but not impossible. We must contend with the institutions, structures, practices, and conventions that people produce, reproduce, and transform. Human meanings and intentions are worked out within the frameworks of these social structures—structures that are invisible, but nonetheless real. In other words, social phenomena such as language, culture, and power exist in the world and exert strong influences over human activities because most people construe them in common ways. Things that are believed become real and can be inquired into.

Understanding the significance of a comprehensive understanding of lived experiences, there have been various calls in the literature for more qualitative research to better understand culturally competent/congruent care,[14,15] social justice issues in animal welfare,[16] and student learning experiences.[9,17] Moreover, qualitative research has long been known as an avenue for giving voice to those often unheard, prioritizing and honoring those voices, and a methodology that allows for more emancipatory, humanizing, liberating research.[3,4,18–23]

Consequently, there has been a notable increase in the publication of qualitative studies in medical and related journals, reflecting its growing significance in human medicine.[24] Medicine encompasses more than just quantitative science, it is also an interpretive art.[3,25] It is vital to probe into the social interactions inherent in health care, which can be systematically explored through qualitative methods.[3,26] This methodology can provide vital insights into the social, emotional, and experiential dimensions of health care.[3]

Just as clinicians integrate various types of information to form clinical judgments, employing complementary research methodologies can enhance our understanding of diverse health issues.[3,27–31] If conducted appropriately, it can additionally ensure that certain voices that have traditionally gone unheard have a platform. This approach is invaluable in illuminating complex human elements that quantitative methods might overlook.

While qualitative research offers a promising path for investigation, it is important to recognize that the field of research itself is built on a foundation that includes systemic racism. The construction of knowledge has long been a battleground where power is asserted: historically, elites have controlled and manipulated knowledge to shape a social imaginary that defines what is considered valid knowledge. To truly commit to the principles of diversity, equity, and inclusion, we must confront and understand the ways in which research has marginalized cultures, communities, and individuals.

Utilizing fundamentally different approaches such as CBPR, which is recognized for its role in promoting health equity by being community-based and often community-directed, can be a transformative step. This approach is not just about placing research in a community setting, but actively involving the community in the research process to ensure that it serves their needs and reflects their values.

Moving forward, we need to reimagine research as an emancipatory and humanizing endeavor. By adopting research orientations that are liberating, we can begin to rectify past injustices and contribute to the creation of a research landscape that upholds the true tenets of diversity, equity, and inclusion.

UNDERSTANDING EPISTEMIC VIOLENCE

To reimagine research, we must first understand the harm caused by research, known by terms such as epistemic silencing, epistemic injustice, and epistemic violence. In this context, epistemic refers to knowledge and the measure of its validation and "other" refers to those that are marginalized by a larger portion of the population and who often maintain limited rights within society.[32] Julieta Paredes, who among many other things is a decolonial feminist activist, has written that it is self-evident that knowledge creation is both a political practice and a collective enterprise.[33] Substantiating Paredes, Dotson has theorized epistemologies not only determine what is considered knowledge but that, "They also generate ordered sets of steps for normative practices that are constrained and licensed by what that epistemic system deems knowledge."[34] As outlined by Berenstain, we must acknowledge and understand that "The construction of knowledge has been a space for power struggles: knowledge has been controlled and manipulated by elites and has served to create a social imaginary of what knowledge is. The body of knowledge: male. The color of knowledge: white. The territories of knowledge: western Europe. The place of knowledge: the academy. Everything and everyone that is outside of these whimsied parameters has historically fought to be recognized as knowledge and as knowing subjects."[35] It is vital that we, as researchers and consumers of research, understand that the western academic world is dominated by colonial White supremacy and that these institutions uphold conceptual traditions that reliably produce epistemic oppression under the guise of objectivity, neutrality, and the faithful application of disciplinary knowledge.[35]

Once this is understood, we can start to conceptualize epistemic violence and, consequently, how to avoid perpetuating this kind of harm.

Perez defines epistemic violence as, "The notion of epistemic violence refers to the different ways in which violence is exercised in relation to the production, circulation and recognition of knowledge: the denial of epistemic agency for certain subjects, the unacknowledged exploitation of their epistemic resources, their objectification, among many others."[36] While violence may initially seem like an exaggerated and dramatic term to use, it is denoted in the literature as a "slow violence" that "occurs gradually and out of sight, a violence of delayed destruction that is dispersed across time and space, an attritional violence that is typically not viewed as violence at all."[37] Contrary to what we typically view as violence, epistemic violence has the characteristics of being gradual and cumulative, difficult to attribute to a particular agent, and imperceptible to many, frequently including its own victims.[36]

In Bunch's 2015 study, they classify epistemic violence into 3 separate categories: discriminatory, testimonial, and distributive.[32]

- Discriminatory epistemic violence: This refers to the dehumanization of marginalized groups, often conceptualized as the "other." It occurs when a dominant group perceives the out-groups as inherently and morally inferior, effectively relegating them to a subhuman status. This perception excludes them from the dominant group's moral and ethical considerations.[38]
- Testimonial epistemic violence: This form of epistemic injustice manifests in 2 ways: diminished credibility and silencing. Diminished credibility occurs when the listener's prejudice leads them to devalue or dismiss the testimony of a marginalized individual, the "other," regardless of their expertise or the validity of their contributions. This prejudicial assessment undermines the speaker's authority and perpetuates their marginalization.[39]
- Distributive epistemic violence: This form of epistemic injustice involves the systematic denial of resources to marginalized groups. It is particularly evident in the withholding of educational opportunities, both within and about these communities.

Having explored the various forms of epistemic violence, including discriminatory, testimonial, and distributive, it becomes crucial to consider methodologies that mitigate these harms within the research process. A foundational approach in this regard is CBPR.

COMMUNITY-BASED PARTICIPATORY RESEARCH

CBPR has long established itself as an avenue for increasing equity as its orientation is community-based, often community-directed, as opposed to just conducted within a community.[21,22] Community in this context is defined as "a group of people with diverse characteristics who are linked by social ties, share common perspectives, and engage in joint action in geographical locations or settings."[40] The context of community has been identified as an important determinant of health outcomes.[40] In the realm of research design and implementation, involving the subjects under study in the research process is increasingly recognized as transformative. This participation not only addresses the complexities inherent in understanding diverse experiences but also acts as a powerful tool for fostering social change.[41,42] Meta-analyses of community-based research and involvement of participants have demonstrated a positive impact on community participants and have led to better-informed science.[41,43] The literature also suggests that health care professionals can benefit from reflecting on how these research methods align with their fields.[44] By understanding this congruence, they can leverage these methods to unlock their profession's emancipatory potential and utilize their professional strengths to bolster the research process.[44] The field of public health provides substantial evidence that simply disseminating study results and instructing individuals on how to apply this information leads to minimal behavioral change.[45] In contrast, participatory research—collaborative investigations conducted by scientists and community members—has resurged in recent decades as an effective alternative. This approach, which contrasts with the traditional top–down model of expert guidance to practitioners or communities, ensures that research outcomes are both relevant and practical, thereby increasing the likelihood that they will be implemented effectively.[45,46] Compared to traditional research approaches, this participatory model necessitates a fundamentally different relationship between researchers and participants, with the latter becoming coresearchers. Achieving this dynamic can be challenging due to the marginalized status of the participants. It requires researchers to be openly self-aware about their own values, priorities, and interpretations of the findings.[44,47]

CBPR is defined in the textbook *Community-Based Participatory Research for Health: Advancing Social and Health Equity*, "CBPR embraces collaborative efforts among community, academic, and other stakeholders who gather and use research and data to build on the strengths and priorities of the community for multilevel strategies to improve health and social equity."[22] They further clarify that CBPR should not be referred to or seen as research method, but an orientation or fundamentally different approach to research.[22] Central to CBPR and similar emancipatory research orientations is the commitment to disrupt the power dynamic between researcher and researched, working to eradicate the distinction between who does the studying and who get studied. This is an intrinsically decolonial action, to move from "studying about to thinking with."[18,22,48]

An important tool for ensuring equality within the research process in utilizing community advisory boards (CABs), which is composed of community members who share a common identity, history, symbols and language, and culture.[49,50] CABs should be involved in all the different aspects of the study, including problem identification, participant recruitment, research monitoring (including retention and follow-up), and dissemination of study findings.[49,51] It is vital that the CAB is actively connected to diverse people in their communities and empowered to function in ways that are meaningful to their communities.[40,52–54] Furthermore, it has been advised in the literature[49,55–58] that CABs are involved during informed consent of research participants and throughout the research process.

While a comprehensive exploration of CBPR and its approaches is beyond the scope of this article, the provided references offer excellent resources for further study. We now shift our focus to perspectives on emancipatory, humanizing, and liberatory research approaches.

EMANCIPATORY, HUMANIZING, AND LIBERATORY APPROACHES

Emancipatory, humanizing, and liberatory approaches to research are essential and must be integrated into any research methodology to prevent the perpetuation of harm to communities categorized as "other." While these approaches are deeply interconnected, they each hold unique characteristics. We will begin by defining each approach clearly. Following that, we will explore the broader implications of applying these approaches in research practices.

Emancipatory research is a research perspective of producing knowledge that can be of benefit to disadvantaged people.[59] It is the process of producing knowledge that has a meaningful practical outcome for those disadvantaged people, can be of benefit to them, and aims to empower its research participants.[23,59] Emancipatory research originated within the disability community, guided by the principle "nothing about us, without us."[60] This approach was developed as a form of political action to shift control of research processes to the communities being studied, ensuring they have a central role in guiding and informing the research that affects them.

Barnes describes the key characteristics of emancipatory disability research as accountability, social model of disability, the problem of objectivity, the choice of methods, the role of experience, and meaningful practical outcomes.[23] While these are specific to disability research, the core principles are transferrable to working with any disadvantaged community and are a useful perspective to look at issues through.

Humanizing research is predicated on the nurturing of relationships of care and dignity among researchers and participants, which can frame research practices such as fieldwork, participant observation, and interviewing.[19,61] These practices help researchers unlearn harmful research practices that engage participants as sites of exploitation and instead consider ways to give to and learn from participants.[19]

Liberatory research is freedom focused and seeks to acknowledge the individual and communal worth of those deemed "other." This approach has the power to emancipate minoritized populations from prescribed narratives of pain and damage in the literature and in society at large.[19]

In their seminal paper, Savage and colleagues[19] challenge the qualitative research community to shift their frameworks and abandon research practices that perpetuate harm and pain. They emphasize the necessity of adopting humanizing and liberatory approaches when conducting research involving racially and ethnically minoritized youth. To support this shift, they provide specific antioppressive strategies and recommendations for researchers working with these communities. While their focus is on youth, the principles and strategies outlined are universally applicable to research involving any disadvantaged communities, promoting broader adoption of these critical approaches.

Savage and colleagues[19] advocate for an end to damage-centered research, which, although it documents the impacts of oppressive structures on racially/ethnically minoritized youth, tends to pathologize these groups by defining them solely through their struggles.[62] To counteract these 1 dimensional portrayals of such youth as broken or deficient, they urge qualitative researchers to expand their focus. This includes highlighting the hopes, desires, agency, and resistance of these groups to ensure a more comprehensive and nuanced representation of their lived experiences, capturing both their challenges and triumphs.

Strategies to approaching and conceptualizing humanizing and liberatory qualitative research advocated by Savage and colleagues[19] emphasize treating racially/ethnically minoritized youth as knowledgeable partners in research that impacts them. By collaborating with participants, researchers can recognize and engage with their humanity, rather than merely viewing them as subjects of study. This involves soliciting participants' input on the questions to be asked, the insights they believe should be pursued, and the data they prefer to remain confidential. Such participatory methods help shift away from extractive, deficit-focused research, promoting a more nuanced and respectful approach that honors participants' complex human experiences.

It is also crucial for research questions to adopt a strengths-based perspective. For example, rather than a deficit-based approach that might ask, "Why are low-income students retained at lower rates?" or "Why are they less engaged on campus?," a strengths-based approach reframes these questions to highlight positive outcomes and agency. Questions could include, "What institutional services do low-income students find most supportive during their college experience?" or "Which campus activities engage low-income students the most?" This method does not overlook the challenges faced by these communities but shifts the focus from their deficits to their strengths and successes, promoting a more balanced and empowering inquiry.[63]

Engaging in liberatory and humanizing research requires challenging the dominant logics and paradigms that shape interactions with minoritized communities. This includes scrutinizing institutional structures like Institutional Review Boards (IRBs), which do not necessarily prevent the "vulnerabilization" of these groups. This term of "vulnerabilization" describes how oppressive, exploitative, and deceitful research practices and policies render groups vulnerable.[64] Critically, IRBs, while established to protect against historical research abuses, often do not address the perpetuation of oppressive and extractive research methods. As Stewart points out, protections are inadequate against research that reinforces oppressive norms.[64] Therefore, qualitative researchers should develop their own internal protocols to mitigate potential harms, including those that institutional safeguards fail to prevent. Researchers need to critically assess how their studies may contribute to or combat systemic injustices, ensuring their study contributes positively to the communities involved. Savage and colleagues provide important questions for antioppressive researchers to consider, including[19]

- What deficit-centered and damage-centered assumptions do I hold about my participants?
- What are the sources of these assumptions?
- In what ways have these assumptions informed my approach (eg, problem formulation, research design, and theoretic orientation) to the study?
- What steps can I take to remediate such assumptions and reduce harm in the research process?
- What is my personal and professional responsibility to the populations and communities I aim to study?
- In what ways have I centered and engaged racially/ethnically minoritized youth in the research process beyond data collection?
- How will I honor and respect the stories and other forms of data that are shared with me through the research process?
- How will I use what is generated from this research to improve the material conditions of the population I am studying?

Savage and colleagues[19] additionally provide 2 tables that present a comparison between 2 approaches to qualitative research. The following table, adapted from their study, outlines the distinct characteristics of damage and deficit-centered qualitative research alongside the principles of humanizing and liberatory qualitative research[19] (**Table 1**).

Table 1
Approaches to qualitative research

Damage and Deficit-centered Qualitative Research	Humanizing and Liberatory Qualitative Research
Stigmatizes and portrays communities as deficient	Recognizes and values participants as complex and knowledgeable
Perpetuates negative myths about marginalized communities	Debunks myths and highlights community resilience and agency
Often excludes participant involvement in research processes	Actively involves participants in all research stages
May result in feelings of embarrassment and inadequacy	Fosters affirmation, belonging, and positive well-being

Data from Savage SS, Johnson RM, Kenney AJ, Haynes DD. Perspectives on Humanizing and Liberatory Qualitative Research with Racially/Ethnically Minoritized Youth. Healthcare (Basel). 2021;9(10):1317. doi:10.3390/healthcare9101317

To conduct qualitative research from an emancipatory, humanizing, and liberatory approach, qualitative researchers must cultivate a critical consciousness and question the prevailing logics of traditional methodologies. This process requires embracing learning, unlearning, and cultural humility. Researchers should collaboratively design studies with the communities involved, prioritize their experiential knowledge, and move away from outdated theories that emphasize deficits. It is crucial to practice critical reflexivity, put the well-being of participants first, and ground research in transformative epistemologies aimed at dismantling oppressive systems.[19]

SUMMARY

In conclusion, this article has highlighted the valuable role of qualitative research in advancing diversity, equity, and inclusion. By delineating the nuances between qualitative and quantitative methodologies, we have identified the unique strengths and weaknesses of qualitative approaches. These insights emphasize the necessity for qualitative research in capturing the complex, lived experiences of diverse populations and in addressing social issues that are often obscured by quantitative methods.

Moreover, we have explored the concept of epistemic violence and the importance of adopting research methodologies and approaches that prevent the perpetuation of harm. CBPR, along with emancipatory, humanizing, and liberatory approaches, exemplifies how the research process can be transformed to empower participants and begin to rectify historical biases.

Ultimately, qualitative research is not just a methodological choice but a relevant tool that can help reshape our understanding of the world and the field of veterinary medicine. It invites us to rethink the foundations of scientific inquiry traditionally utilized in our field and to embrace a new paradigm that values and prioritizes diversity, equity, and inclusion. This article serves as a call to researchers and practitioners alike to adopt these transformative approaches, thereby enriching the scientific community and the broader society it serves.

DISCLOSURE

Declaration of artificial intelligence (AI) and AI-assisted technologies in the writing process. During the preparation of this study the author used ChatGPT4 in order to improve readability. After using this tool, the author reviewed and edited the content as needed and takes full responsibility for the content of the publication.

REFERENCES

1. Tenny S, Brannan JM, Brannan GD. Qualitative study. In: StatPearls. StatPearls Publishing; 2024. Available at: http://www.ncbi.nlm.nih.gov/books/NBK470395/. [Accessed 17 April 2024].
2. Foley G, Timonen V. Using grounded theory method to capture and analyze health care experiences. Health Serv Res 2015;50(4):1195–210.
3. Giacomini MK, Cook DJ, Group for the EBMW. Users' guides to the medical literature: XXIII. Qualitative Research in Health Care A. Are the Results of the Study Valid? JAMA 2000;284(3):357–62.
4. Miles MB, Huberman AM, Saldana J. Qualitative data analysis: a methods Sourcebook. Thousand Oaks, CA: SAGE Publications; 2013.
5. Devers KJ. How will we know "good" qualitative research when we see it? Beginning the dialogue in health services research. Health Serv Res 1999;34(5 Pt 2):1153–88.

6. Lived Experience, In: Given L.M., editor. The SAGE encyclopedia of qualitative research methods, 2008, SAGE Publications, Inc.; Thousand Oaks, CA. 490.
7. Ryan S, Ziebland S. On interviewing people with pets: reflections from qualitative research on people with long-term conditions. Sociol Health Illness 2015;37(1): 67–80.
8. Charles N, Davies CA. My family and other animals: pets as kin. Socio Res Online 2008;13(5):13–26.
9. Jafarian S, Akpek E, Reinhard CL, et al. A qualitative analysis of clinical year veterinary student journal entries for a shelter medicine rotation. Front Vet Sci 2022; 9. Available at: https://www.frontiersin.org/articles/10.3389/fvets.2022.858419. [Accessed 31 August 2022].
10. Chapman A, Hadfield M, Chapman C. Qualitative research in healthcare: an introduction to grounded theory using thematic analysis. J R Coll Physicians Edinb 2015;45(3):201–5.
11. Mays N, Pope C. Qualitative research in health care: assessing quality in qualitative research. BMJ 2000;320. Available at: https://www-jstor-org.proxy.library.upenn.edu/stable/25186737?pq-origsite=summon&seq=1#metadata_info_tab_contents. [Accessed 19 March 2020].
12. MacQueen KM, McLellan E, Kay K, et al. Codebook development for team-based qualitative analysis. CAM Journal 1998;10(2):31–6.
13. Tesch R. Qualitative research : analysis types and software tools/. Bristol, PA: Falmer Press; 1990.
14. Handtke O, Schilgen B, Mösko M. Culturally competent healthcare – A scoping review of strategies implemented in healthcare organizations and a model of culturally competent healthcare provision. PLoS One 2019;14(7):e0219971.
15. Schim SM, Doorenbos A, Benkert R, et al. Culturally congruent care: putting the puzzle together. J Transcult Nurs 2007;18(2):103–10.
16. Jenkins JL, Rudd ML. Decolonizing animal welfare through a social justice framework. Front Vet Sci 2022;8. Available at: https://www.frontiersin.org/articles/10.3389/fvets.2021.787555. [Accessed 17 August 2022].
17. Pandhi N, Gaines M, Deci D, et al. Broadening medical students' exposure to the range of illness experiences: a pilot curriculum focused on depression education. Acad Med 2020;95(1):72.
18. Milián Bernal D. Challenging methodologies: deploying liberatory epistemologies to unlock creative research practices. Qual Res 2023. https://doi.org/10.1177/14687941231176938. 14687941231176938.
19. Savage SS, Johnson RM, Kenney AJ, et al. Perspectives on humanizing and liberatory qualitative research with racially/ethnically minoritized youth. Healthcare (Basel) 2021;9(10):1317.
20. Hinkelmann M, Mendívil ER. When research on Epistemic Violence becomes violent. Towards a dialectical materialist critique 2016.
21. Sande A van de, Schwartz K. Research for social justice: a community-based participatory approach. Halifax, Nova Scotia: Fernwood Publishing Company Ltd; 2017.
22. Wallerstein N, Duran B, Oetzel JG, et al. Community-based participatory research for health: advancing social and health equity. Hoboken, NJ: John Wiley & Sons; 2017.
23. Barnes C. 'Emancipatory disability research': project or process? J Res Spec Educ Needs 2002;2(1).
24. Harding G, Gantley M. Qualitative methods: beyond the cookbook. Fam Pract 1998;15(1):76–9.

25. Battista RN, Hodge MJ, Vineis P. Medicine, practice and guidelines: The uneasy juncture of science and art. J Clin Epidemiol 1995;48(7):875–80.
26. Hughes J, Sharrock W. The interpretive alternative. In: The philosophy of social research. New York, NY: Longman; 1990. p. 89–112.
27. Rosenfield PL. The potential of transdisciplinary research for sustaining and extending linkages between the health and social sciences. Soc Sci Med 1992; 35(11):1343–57.
28. Stange KC, Zyzanski SJ. Integrating qualitative and quantitative research methods. Fam Med 1989;21(6):448–51.
29. Reconcilable Differences. The Marriage of Qualitative and Quantitative Methods - Paula N Goering, David L Streiner. 1996. Available at: https://journals.sagepub.com/doi/abs/10.1177/070674379604100804. [Accessed 21 April 2024].
30. Magnier K, Wang R, Dale VHM, et al. Enhancing clinical learning in the workplace: a qualitative study. Vet Rec 2011;169(26):682.
31. Patton MQ. Enhancing the quality and credibility of qualitative analysis. Health Serv Res 1999;34(5 Pt 2):1189–208.
32. Bunch A. Epistemic violence in the process of othering: real-world applications and moving forward. Scholarly Undergraduate Research Journal at Clark (SURJ) 2015;1(1). Available at: https://commons.clarku.edu/surj/vol1/iss1/2.
33. Paredes J. Hilando fino desde el feminismo indigena comunitario. In: Aproximaciones Criticas a Las Practicas Teorico-Politicas Del Feminismo Latinoamericano. Vol 1. 1st ed. Y. Espinosa Miñoso (Comp); 2010:117-120.
34. Dotson K. Tales from an apostate. Phil Issues 2019;29(1):69–83.
35. Berenstain N, Dotson K, Paredes J, et al. Epistemic oppression, resistance, and resurgence. Contemp Polit Theor 2022;21(2):283–314.
36. Pérez M. Epistemic violence: reflections between the invisible and the ignorable. El lugar sin límites 2019;1(1):81–98.
37. Nixon R. Slow violence and the environmentalism of the poor. Harvard University Press; 2011. Available at: https://www.degruyter.com/document/doi/10.4159/harvard.9780674061194/html. [Accessed 21 April 2024].
38. Maoz I, McCauley C. Threat, dehumanization, and support for retaliatory aggressive policies in asymmetric conflict. J Conflict Resolut 2008;52(1):93–116.
39. Fricker M. Epistemic justice as a condition of political freedom? Synthese 2013; 190(7):1317–32.
40. MacQueen KM, McLellan E, Metzger DS, et al. What is community? An evidence-based definition for participatory public health. Am J Publ Health 2001;91(12): 1929–38.
41. Burks-Abbott G, Gannaway A, Szarkowski A, et al. Virtual advocacy: lived experience takes center stage during and after pandemic. Developmental Disabilities Network Journal 2021;1(2).
42. Mertens DM. Transformative paradigm: mixed methods and social justice. J Mix Methods Res 2007;1(3):212–25.
43. Ortiz K, Nash J, Shea L, et al. Partnerships, processes, and outcomes: a health equity–focused scoping meta-review of community-engaged scholarship. Annu Rev Publ Health 2020;41:177–99.
44. Kramer-Roy D. Using participatory and creative methods to facilitate emancipatory research with people facing multiple disadvantage: a role for health and care professionals. Disabil Soc 2015;30(8):1207–24.
45. Green LW, Mercer SL. Can public health researchers and agencies reconcile the push from funding bodies and the pull from communities? Am J Publ Health 2001; 91(12):1926–9.

46. Park P, Brydon-Miller M, Hall B, et al. Voices of change : participatory research in the United States and Canada. Bergin & Garvey; 1993. Available at: https://lccn.loc.gov/92042898. [Accessed 21 April 2024].
47. Barton L. Emancipatory research and disabled people: some observations and questions. Educ Rev 2005;57(3):317–27.
48. Mignolo WD, Walsh CE. On decoloniality: concepts, analytics, praxis. Durham, NC: Duke University Press; 2018.
49. Strauss RP, Sengupta S, Quinn SC, et al. The role of community advisory boards: involving communities in the informed consent process. Am J Publ Health 2001; 91(12):1938–43.
50. Israel BA, Checkoway B, Schulz A, et al. Health Education and Community Empowerment: Conceptualizing and Measuring Perceptions of Individual, Organizational, and Community Control. Health Educ Behav 1994;21(2). https://doi.org/10.1177/109019819402100203.
51. Strauss T. Community advisory board investigator relationship in community-based research. In: King NMP, Henderson GE, Stein J, editors. Beyond regulations: ethics in human subjects research. Chapel Hill, NC: University of North Carolina Press; 1999. p. 94–101.
52. Conway T, Hu TC, Harrington T. Setting health priorities: community boards accurately reflect the preferences of the community's residents. J Commun Healthc 1997;22(1):57–68.
53. Jewkes R, Murcott A. Community representatives: Representing the "community". Soc Sci Med 1998;46(7):843–58.
54. Bond MA, Keys CB. Empowerment, diversity, and collaboration: promoting synergy on community boards. Am J Community Psychol 1993;21(1):37–57.
55. AIDS *vaccine advocacy coalition. 8 Years and counting*, 1999, What Will Speed Development of an AIDS Vaccine? Presented at; Washington, DC. Available at: https://avac.org/resource/report/1999-avac-report-8-years-and-counting-what-will-speed-the-development-of-an-aids-vaccine/. (Accessed 21 April 2024).
56. Barry M. Ethical Considerations of Human Investigation in Developing Countries: The AIDS Dilemma. BRL:KIE/27409 1988. Available at: https://repository.library.georgetown.edu/handle/10822/731670. [Accessed 21 April 2024].
57. Levine RJ. Ethics and regulation of clinical research. New Haven, CT: Yale University Press; 1988.
58. Melton GB, Levine RJ, Koocher GP, et al. Community consultation in socially sensitive research: lessons from clinical trials of treatments for AIDS. In: Schüklenk U, editor. AIDS: society, ethics and law. London, UK: Routledge; 2001. p. 573–81.
59. Noel LA. Promoting an emancipatory research paradigm in Design Education and Practice. DRS Biennial Conference Series. 2016. Available at: https://dl.designresearchsociety.org/drs-conference-papers/drs2016/researchpapers/157.
60. Charlton JI. Nothing about us without us: disability oppression and empowerment. Oakland, CA: University of California Press; 1998.
61. Paris D. "A friend who understand fully": notes on humanizing research in a multiethnic youth community. Int J Qual Stud Educ 2011;24(2):137–49.
62. Tuck E. Suspending damage: a letter to communities. Harv Educ Rev 2009;79(3): 409–28.
63. Harper SR. An anti-deficit achievement framework for research on students of color in STEM. N Dir Inst Res 2010. https://doi.org/10.1002/ir.362.
64. Stewart DL. Performing goodness in qualitative research methods. Int J Qual Stud Educ 2022;35(1):58–70.

Understanding Implicit Bias and Its Impact in Veterinary Medicine

Jean-Yin Tan, DVM, MBA[a,*], Katherine Fogelberg, DVM, PhD[b]

KEYWORDS

• Implicit bias • Stereotype • Diversity • Inclusion • Equity • Racism

KEY POINTS

- Implicit biases are biases one is unwilling to admit to, yet they influence behavior in ways that impact the workplace experience.
- Implicit bias influences choice of veterinary career and limits success within a chosen career pathway.
- Discrimination in the veterinary workplace is pervasive and has a negative impact that is responsible for financial loss.
- Implicit bias influences client communication and patient-care.
- Strategies can be employed to acknowledge implicit bias and foster behavioral change.

AUTHORS' NOTE

As women of color who have been part of this profession for several decades, we bring our own perspectives, experiences, and interpretations of the literature to this topic. We do not profess to speak for all women of color, all women, or the "all" of any other group to which we feel we belong or into which others might put us. This article relies on the literature, as it should, but we wanted to provide a little bit of our backgrounds in acknowledgment of our own biases up front.

INTRODUCTION AND HISTORY

In the late 1990s, a group of social psychologists developed the Implicit Association Test (IAT), which was intended to measure implicit biases. Conducted online, it has now been taken by millions; most forms of the IAT focus on race, although some focus on disability, weight, and others. Many may be familiar with the IAT; perhaps even taken 1 or more of them and been potentially surprised at the results. For those

[a] University of Calgary, CSB 112N, 11877-85th Street Northwest, Calgary, Alberta T3R 1J3 Canada; [b] Thrive Pet Healthcare, 211 Walter Seaholm Drive, #200 Austin, TX 78701, USA
* Corresponding author.
E-mail address: jeanyin.tan@ucalgary.ca

Vet Clin Small Anim 54 (2024) 813–824
https://doi.org/10.1016/j.cvsm.2024.06.005 vetsmall.theclinics.com
0195-5616/24/

familiar, the IAT has been an interesting experience; for those in social psychology and other fields; however, it has presented some interesting controversy.

Before diving into the controversy; however, it is important to provide a definition of "implicit bias" and some other important key words or phrases that cannot be ignored in a discussion of this topic, including "explicit bias" and "stereotyping." Currently, implicit bias, also referred to as "unconscious bias," appears to be a rather straightforward concept, though in reality it can be somewhat challenging to define with specificity.[1]

DEFINITIONS AND BACKGROUND

In social psychology, implicit bias is defined through contrasting it with its opposite–explicit bias. Thus, implicit biases are those demonstrated during a task but are not self-reported. In their simplest forms, implicit biases are those we may hold with or without realizing it and are, therefore, unwilling or unable to admit, while explicit biases are those we are willing to admit and that are consciously controlled.[1,2] For example, I may admit that I love dogs and not admit that I actually love cats more, but when dealing with dogs and cats I may exhibit favoritism toward cats, uncovering an implicit bias against dogs.

While implicit bias itself is not necessarily controversial, its conflation with the term "unconscious bias" has become problematic. "Unconscious" carries the connotation that an individual is unaware of their bias(es), and thus, unable to control behaviors that may stem from such an "unconscious" belief or attitude; it can be thought of as a scale, from "unconscious" (meaning wholly unaware of, therefore behaviors are uncontrolled), to "implicit" (aware of but unwilling to admit to, therefore behaviors are controllable), to "explicit" (aware of, admits to, and actively works to control behaviors) – including stereotyping. A "stereotype" is defined by the Oxford Languages dictionary as "a widely held but fixed and oversimplified image or idea of a particular type of person or thing".[3] To illustrate further, Greenwald and Krieger explain that "A social *stereotype* is a mental association between a social group or category and a trait".[4(p949)] Greenwald (one of the originators of the IAT) and Krieger go on to explain that stereotypes may be associated with favorable or unfavorable traits within a group.[4] The difference between stereotypes and attitudes is that in a stereotype, the trait of the group is expressed upon the individual, whereas in an attitude, there is an evaluation of that trait's positive or negative perception.[4] That is, if one expressed a stereotype of pop music artists, they might say "all female pop artists are skinny," (a perceived trait); if they were expressing an attitude toward pop artists, they might say "all female pop artists are stuck up" (an evaluation of the group).

The relationship between implicit biases and stereotypes is an easy–and important–one to identify. While the aforementioned example aptly illustrates the connection between explicit biases and stereotypes, there are multitudes of examples demonstrating implicit bias and stereotypes. For example, many of us may profess the value of having women in high-ranking leadership roles while still viewing identical credentials of male and female candidates differently; a woman and mother to a toddler may be viewed as less capable of doing a job than a man and father to a toddler. This likely comes from the common stereotype of "female as primary caregiver," often resulting from an implicit bias that women are more nurturing than men.

Unconscious bias being viewed synonymously with implicit bias has led many to argue that stereotyping and other behaviors resulting from biases may be excusable because the individual is unaware of their biases and how they influence behaviors. But studies have demonstrated that equating "unconscious" with "implicit" bias essentially provides individuals an "excuse" to discriminate–or at least something to blame their discrimination on without having to take moral ownership of their behavior. In one study, for example, it was found that-

When participants learned about acts of racial discrimination that were not explained by any psychologic theory, they made the most severe moral judgments. When the discrimination was explained as a result of automatic bias that was unconscious but difficult to control, their moral judgments were not much changed. But when they learned that the discrimination resulted from unconscious bias–an attitude that the agent did not know existed–their moral judgments were significantly more lenient.[5(p285)]

This aligns with Greenwald and Krieger's observation that "The term 'bias'...denotes a displacement of people's responses along a continuum of possible judgments".[4] Additionally, "*Implicit biases* are discriminatory biases based on implicit attitudes or implicit stereotypes. Implicit biases are especially intriguing, and also especially problematic, because they can produce behavior that diverges from a person's avowed or endorsed beliefs or principles"–which may also include explicit biases.[4(p951)]

This leads us back to that IAT. With millions of data points, it has often been cited as evidence that implicit bias is real. No one is arguing that implicit bias is not real. Rather, there is a concern that conflating *implicit bias* with *unconscious bias* insinuates that associated behaviors cannot be controlled and, therefore, responsibility cannot be assigned. Selmi does an excellent job of exploring this fallacy and the impacts this conflation can have legally.[1]

Perhaps in anticipation of these concerns, Greenwald and Krieger published a meta-analysis of the IAT demonstrating that it and parallel explicit measures displayed predictive validity with regard to behavior.[4] In general, predictive validity was greater for the self-reported (explicit) measures than for IAT measure, but "within a critical group of studies that focused on prejudicial attitudes and stereotypes–in other words, within the studies of implicit bias–*predictive validity was significantly greater for the IAT measures*."[4(p954)] Additionally, in socially sensitive situations, the implicit measures of bias had "relatively greater validity than explicit measures".[4(p954)] And, "implicit measures have relatively greater validity in predicting spontaneous behaviors such as eye contact, seating distance, and other such actions that communicate social warmth or discomfort".[4(p955)] From this assessment, they concluded that "the dominant interpretation of this evidence is that implicit attitudinal biases are especially important in influencing nondeliberate or spontaneous discriminatory behaviors".[4(p961)]

That implicit bias is more akin to stereotyping appears to have been overlooked for decades, as "the founders of the IAT routinely refer to implicit biases as stereotypes and have for many years".[1(p37)] Perhaps the move to equating "implicit bias" with "stereotype" may encounter some issue in future, but currently it seems reasonable to take into consideration, especially since the IAT has come under increased scrutiny and criticism within social psychology, in contrast to the enthusiastic reception it received from other professions and the public. In fact, in 2016, several social psychologists affiliated with the IAT worked on a paper that "found 'little to no evidence' that changes in implicit bias led to changes in either behavior or explicit bias"– supporting the very weak link found between implicit bias scores and behavior.[1(p961)]

Ultimately, we cannot take those who deny intent to discriminate as accurate representations of an individual's thoughts; one may actively and consciously discriminate against someone for some reason that, when asked about their decision–would deny they actively and consciously did so. There are multiple reasons people do this, but in the end the reason does not matter. What matters is that what people say, what people do, and what people think are not always aligned, so defining implicit bias as unconscious and uncontrollable may, in many ways, be doing the opposite of what it was intended to do. That is, it is providing a shield for many to continue overt and covert discrimination rather than making us more aware that our actions may be influenced by prejudices and that we should actively work against making judgements or taking actions based on these.

DISCUSSION

Implicit bias within the veterinary field is important to understand because it has the potential to influence those entering and selecting their pathway within the profession, affect workplace satisfaction and progression, and impact client and patient-care.

Implicit Bias and Career Pathway

Implicit bias includes both the attitudes and stereotypes affecting decisions. Agathou and colleagues investigated the influence of stereotypes and implicit bias surrounding career choice within veterinary medicine.[6] Word cloud and sentiment analysis of single adjective descriptions by 665 veterinary students, staff, and professionals revealed strong professional stereotypes, and 82% of participants agreed that stereotypes exist. For example, small animal practitioners were described as caring, friendly, compassionate, kind, and empathetic. In contrast, equine general practitioners were described as posh, arrogant or snobby, and surgeons were described as arrogant. Production animal general practitioners were associated with the males and behavioral medicine associated with females, and prestige was associated with neurology, surgery, and cardiology. Such negative or positive stereotypes may factor in students' career ambitions, as a survey of 261 United Kingdom (UK) graduates found fewer females willing to choose farm animal or equine practice.[7]

Bias may play a role in clinical grading and senior award receipt in veterinary schools. Nelson *and colleagues* found that although female students are overrepresented in the top cohort in the preclinical curriculum, male students are more likely to receive awards than female students.[8] Nonwhite female students in the top quintile were less likely than white female students to receive awards and nonwhite ethnicity was associated with lower grades and lower deciles or quintiles among female students. Thus, implicit bias may play a role in veterinary education, which may then impact a student's choice of career pathway.

Stereotyping within a profession may lead to discrimination within the community, self-selection bias, and limited career aspirations within a field. For example, sexual and gender minorities in human medicine rate their sexual orientation or gender identity as strong influencers of specialty choice and tend to self-select away from specialty prestige when these career choices were inversely related to existing minorities and perceived to be less inclusive.[9] Gloria and Hird's study supports this premise, finding that racial and ethnic minority students have lower career decision-making self-efficacy, meaning that they have low expectations for being placed in their chosen occupation and their acceptance into the workforce because of the predominantly white field.[10] They also had higher anxiety relative to career decision-making due to less perceived control and influence over potential work environments. There also appears to be a relationship between marginalized identities and career mobility. McGinn and Milkman followed personnel over 5 years at a large law firm and found that higher numbers of same-sex superiors improved junior professionals' career mobility while there are mobility costs for those with higher proportions of same-sex and same-race peers.[11]

Job procurement and successful application to residencies may also be influenced by implicit bias. Studies show that racially identifiable Asian and African American names were up to 40% less likely to receive a call back by small businesses.[12,13] In human medicine, race but not gender is associated with lower odds of admission into orthopedic surgery residency despite equivalent academic metrics.[14] All racial minorities felt a need for additional specialty training and most racial minority residents were less likely to feel they fit in their programs.[15] Minority residents also reported less positive relationships with faculty and peers and were more likely to feel attendings would think worse of them when asked for help, and less likely to feel they could count on their peers for help.

Race similarity and implicit bias may also play a role in mentoring. The similarity-attraction paradigm describes the positive impression and attraction that plays a role due to demographic similarity.[16,17] This phenomenon may help to explain the gender and racial bias in clinical grading and senior award receipt described by Nelson *and colleagues*[8] in veterinary schools, as white male faculty members may disproportionately reward demographically similar veterinary students. Race similarity has a positive effect on mentees seeking out mentors and initiating relationships, with mentees more affected than mentors.[17] This is particularly important when people have strong race dissimilarity biases. For example, white individuals who believe they have experienced reverse discrimination will intentionally avoid mentoring minority mentees.[17]

Given the role that implicit bias and the similarity-attraction paradigm play in selecting career pathway in health care fields, recognizing and addressing these biases throughout the stages of the veterinary profession is important.

Implicit Bias in the Veterinary Workplace

Evidence supports that implicit bias has a significant and negative impact on the American workplace. A study of the data from the United States (US) Equal Employment Opportunity Commission demonstrated that workplace discrimination may be based more on stigma than on worker capability. This work suggested that employers may be implicitly labeling racialized employees as disabled when they are not. It also found that implicit bias against those with perceived disabilities in the workplace, evidenced by significantly more merit resolutions (favorable employee outcomes) for people with perceived disabilities than those with documented disabilities.[18]

Within the veterinary profession, Loomans *and colleagues* found that 80% of Dutch equine practitioners surveyed felt that occupational disability could significantly impact professional relationships within the practice but rarely resulted in changes.[19] Smits *and colleagues* postulated that people with autistic spectrum conditions may self-select into the profession (due to technical skill, hyper-focus, curiosity, and attention to detail) and found that mental well-being for autistic veterinarians was well below veterinary and adult norms, with psychosocial working conditions (demands, control, managerial support, peer support, relationships, role, and change) accounting for 44% of the variance.[20]

The impact of implicit bias also affects the workplace overall. Carr *and colleagues* found that a high sense of belonging is associated with a 56% increase in performance, 50% decrease in turnover, 75% decrease in sick days, 167% increase in willingness to promote the company, double the raises, 18 times the promotions, and the equivalent of $52 million savings for a 10000-person company.[21] They also found that people in a virtual ball-toss game who were not thrown the ball often were less likely to work hard for a team task, even though this meant sacrificing some of their individual cut of the earnings.[21] When told earnings were individual, they worked as hard as those who were thrown the ball often. Perhaps most remarkably, having even 1 ally (1 bot throwing the ball to the participant while others ignored them) protected group performance.

When implicit bias affects one's sense of belonging in the workplace, it not a far leap that this might decrease overall productivity of the team and organization.

Unfortunately, despite the impact of sense of belonging on productivity and health and well-being, discrimination in the veterinary workplace is pervasive. For example, LGBTQ + veterinarians have higher prevalence of suicidal ideation and attempted suicide than other veterinarians, who already have higher suicide rates than the public.[22]

Discrimination is also well-documented within veterinary education. A survey of veterinary schools in the UK found 36% of veterinary students perceived discriminatory behavior, most commonly from supervising veterinarians (39%), but only 14% of the students reported it.[23] Another UK veterinary student survey found that 77% of students' animal husbandry placements demonstrated discrimination; 38% of the discrimination related to gender and 16% to ethnicity.[24] In a qualitative study of ethnic diversity and veterinary student experiences, discrimination led to minority stress on top of increased financial and family pressures.[25] All students shared stories of racism and discrimination, and many noted difficulties in transitioning to the majority white environment where people who looked like them did not hold career positions they desired.

Women currently make up 65% of the veterinary workforce and 84% of new graduates, yet the gender wage gap persists.[26] Among veterinarians earning over $200000 per year, women earn on average $100000 less than men.[27] The largest study of the state of women in corporate America, with the data from 450000 workers and 900 companies, described 4 myths inhibiting females' workplace progress: Women are less ambitious, the glass ceiling, microaggressions have micro impact, and women want flexible work.[28] Their results contradict these stereotypes; women and men were equally interested in senior leadership roles and there is a missing rung in promotion: 87 women and 72 women of color were promoted for every 100 men. For Black women, only 52 are promoted for every 100 men. Microaggressions made women feel unsafe to take risks, propose new ideas, or raise concerns in the workplace. They were 3 times more likely to consider quitting and 4 times more likely to be burned out. Finally, although 38% of women with children need workplace flexibility, 83% of employees (of both genders) believe they can work better remotely.

Implicit Bias Affecting Clients and Patient-Care

The connection between implicit bias and client and patient-care is most evident in human medical literature. A systematic review found evidence of implicit bias in health care professionals, with racial or ethnic and gender biases most investigated.[29] All studies found a significant relationship between implicit bias and lower quality care. Most studies used the IAT or combined the IAT with another measure and concluded that middle-aged women with coronary heart disease are twice as likely to receive a mental health diagnosis, physician interactions tend to be negatively rated by Black patients and external observers, and nurses show bias toward injecting drug users. One study found that bias made pediatricians more likely to prescribe painkillers to white patients compared to Black patients, with explicit biases associated with treatment recommendations.[30]

Communication is affected by bias and creates health disparities for people. Schut discovered that health providers are less likely to communicate incidental medical findings to patients of color relative to white patients.[31] A systematic review demonstrated that Black patients experience poorer communication, information-giving, participation, and participatory decision-making relative to white patients. It also found that racial concordance is associated with better communication.[32]

While not as robust, literature on the effects of implicit bias on veterinary care does exist. The Brakke management and behavior study identified implicit bias associated with clients and business practices.[33] A split questionnaire (half indicated the client was a "successful young professional" and half indicated "an elderly widow of modest means") asked veterinarians to select a treatment and quote pricing for a highly valued pet with renal failure. The results strongly suggested implicit bias: Twice as many veterinarians recommended the lower level of treatment and quoted the lower mean price to the widow as compared to the young professional.[33]

More recently, Hoffman *and colleagues* explored implicit bias during a virtual shelter medicine rotation.[34] In pre- and post-test surveys relating to a 4-week virtual rotation, students showed increased detection of implicit bias toward pet owners through identification of statements demonstrating such bias. Recognition of such statements reduced their tendency to be judgmental of veterinary clients.

However, community-based primary care veterinary clinics involving First Nations communities in Ontario may perpetuate bias.[35] According to one participant, these initiatives could be "perpetuating white savior stereotypes and other neocolonialist tropes" from lack of understanding and training in cultural bias. Only 22% of students believed they learned about Indigenous cultures by participating in the clinics and there were "repeated calls from several students for more training, with some expressing concern that without this knowledge, harm could be done." Thus, community-based outreach veterinary services highlight the potential for bias affecting client and patient-care, particularly when it comes to implicit biases toward low-income clients and other vulnerable communities. This potential for bias highlights the importance of impact evaluation of programs involving vulnerable communities and a concerted "first, do no harm" approach to community-based practice. [41]

Solutions

Evidence demonstrates that bias plays a role in career determination, workplace satisfaction and safety, and client and patient-care. So how can we mitigate implicit bias within the profession?

Two main strategies exist to combat implicit bias: (1) Conscious recognition of biases and (2) Fostering behavioral change.[36] Transformative learning theory is one approach that educational institutions may take to mitigate implicit bias.[36] Step 1 involves a disorienting experience to help an individual recognize their biases. For example, IAT participation or a video observation of an interaction. Step 2 is critical reflection through self-reflection or large-group discussion, and step 3 is skill acquisition and behavior change through role play or simulated clients.

While the studies on the association of implicit bias with veterinary care are few and far between, and combating bias has little to no research within veterinary medicine, human medical literature has explored how implicit bias can be mitigated. Transformative learning theory (TLT; using critical reflection and dialogue to disrupt assumptions), combined with implicit bias management techniques, are effective in increasing awareness of bias and action in challenging leadership, as well as oneself.[37] Implicit bias recognition and management (IBRM) is a skills-based approach using recognition of implicit bias and skills to address implicit bias. Using IBRM (eg, observation, reflections, IAT, and facilitated discussions) and TLT can improve the skills needed to address bias in the real world.

Fostering diversity and inclusion can also combat bias, as shown by intergroup contact theory, which posits that contact between groups can lead to positive effects if there is equal group status within the situation, common goals, intergroup cooperation, and the support of authorities, law, or custom.[38] Contact with marginalized identities, particularly between equals, has been shown to decrease bias. In one study, over 4000 medical students across the US found 82% of respondents exhibited implicit bias against gay and lesbian individuals versus 46% demonstrating explicit bias.[2] Consistent with intergroup contact theory, positive attitudes developed with increased amount and favorability of contact with individuals. However, while empathy mitigated explicit bias, implicit bias did not improve.

Tackling systemic barriers is important in recognizing and combating bias inherent in the workplace. Field *and colleagues* believe workplace outcomes should be tracked to compare the progress of employees of different genders and race/ethnicity.[28] Inequities should be addressed to recognize and challenge microaggressions; performance reviews and promotions should be de-biased; and work flexibility can improve equity in the workplace. Society is asking companies to do more than share demographics demonstrating they have diversity, resulting in more companies aiming to be fully accountable. The use of data-driven outcomes to measure their progress by instituting accountability infrastructure, diversity, equity, and inclusion infrastructure, tracking progression, measuring well-being through the proportion of the workforce that works when sick, and ensuring that misconduct reports are resolved in a way that satisfies the reporter is increasing.[39] Such policies have evidence that they support marginalized populations. For example, the total number of LGBTA + policies, resources, and gender identity disclosures in the veterinary workplace were associated with job satisfaction and negatively associated with emotional exhaustion.[22] And an equitable workplace that fosters diverse leadership may be particularly effective in breaking down barriers. Those in leadership positions are empowered to create reform by addressing the needs of others with commonalities, catalyzing downstream improvement in systems that reduce minority stress.

Systemic change is important in supporting diversity, equity, inclusion, and belonging, while interpersonal treatment in the workplace is equally important. The earlier example of an ally throwing a virtual ball to an employee protecting group performance demonstrates that microinclusions–brief moments of treatment, especially from those in the dominant group, that clarify and positively influence how others treat themselves in a social context–can improve peoples' experiences in their workplace through increasing a sense of belonging.[40] Evidence supports that both men and women benefit from microinclusions, although women and their anticipated fit in the workplace are affected more positively than men.

SUMMARY

Presented here are definitions of implicit bias, explicit bias, unconscious bias, and stereotypes. Research clearly demonstrates that implicit bias plays a significant role in the veterinary professional's quality of life, and their experiences in turn affect the profession. Definitions were followed by extensive discussion about the impact implicit bias has on individuals' choice of career pathway, workplace experience, and patient-care. Although human medical literature is more robust, it seems reasonable that implicit bias's impacts there can, to some extent, be extrapolated to veterinary medicine.

Some evidence-based suggestions for combating implicit bias were also provided. Like all work involving humans, helping others understand that implicit bias is real, that it affects the experiences of our colleagues, patients, and clients, and that it can be combated are the first steps.

CONCLUSION

It is important to recognize the need for more veterinary-focused research in this area, both to confirm the findings from the human medical literature and to discover any possible unique issues within veterinary medicine. It is also necessary to determine if the solutions found and discussed here are as effective in the veterinary profession as they have been in the human medical profession, and whether there are other ways to mitigate implicit bias's negative impacts.

The work to increase awareness and point out how implicit bias affects our profession is part of why this article was written. The work to combat implicit bias is harder. We have provided some evidence-based suggestions for how to do so with the understanding that implementing such solutions can be difficult. In spite of this, we strongly believe the work is important for a number of reasons, including: (1) it will improve access to the profession and, therefore, increase diversity, (2) it will promote equity and inclusion, (3) it will improve the quality of life for marginalized individuals, (4) patient-care will be positively impacted, and finally, (5) it is the right thing to do. The hard work is continuous and sometimes arduous, but can have positive impacts both tangibly (eg, increased revenues and diversity within the profession) and intangibly (eg, increased quality of life for colleagues, clients, and patients).

Thus, we end with a challenge to our readers: how will you personally work to identify and mitigate your implicit biases, and how will you then use that experience to help others do the same?

CLINICS CARE POINTS

- Recognizing that implicit bias is more akin to stereotyping and is not necessarily unconscious and uncontrollable, empowers a person to actively work against making judgements and to take actions accordingly.
- Implicit bias may affect a career pathway in veterinary and human health care by influencing professional stereotypes, impacting clinical grading and senior award receipt, limiting self-selection into various specialty choices, and may affect mentorship and ultimately job and residency procurement.
- Implicit bias has a negative impact on the workplace by affecting performance, turnover, sick days, and success within a company. Discrimination is documented in veterinary schools and a significant gender wage gap persists in the veterinary workforce.
- Implicit bias is correlated with lower quality patient-care and poorer communication in human medicine.
- Combatting implicit bias in veterinary medicine may include implementing transformative learning theory, fostering diversity and inclusion, and tackling stystemic inequities. Further, improving individual interpersonal treatment through microinclusions can improve the workplace experience.

DISCLOSURE

The authors have nothing to disclose.

REFERENCES

1. Selmi M. The paradox of implicit bias and a plea for a new narrative. Washington, DC: GW Law Faculty Publications & Other Works; 2017. p. 1–41.
2. Burke SE, Dovidio JF, Przedworski JM, et al. Do Contact and Empathy Mitigate Bias Against Gay and Lesbian People Among Heterosexual First-Year Medical Students? A Report From the Medical Student CHANGE Study. Acad Med 2015;90(5):645–51.

3. Oxford Language Dictionary online via Google search. Available at: https://www.google.com/search?q=stereotype&oq=stereotype&gs_lcrp=EgZjaHJvbWUyDAgAEEUYORixAxiABDIGCAEQRRhAMgoIAhAAGLEDGIAEMgoIAxAAGLEDGIAEMgoIBBAAGLEDGIAEMgoIBRAAGLEDGIAEMgoIBhAAGLEDGIAEMgYIBxBFGDzSAQgyNDA2ajBqOagCALACAA&sourceid=chrome&ie=UTF-8. Accessed January 4, 2024.
4. Greenwald AG, Krieger LH. Implicit bias: Scientific foundations. Calif Law Rev 2006;945–67.
5. Cameron CD, Payne BK, Knobe J. Do theories of implicit race bias change moral judgments? Soc Justice Res 2010.
6. Agathou S, Stratis A, Routh J, et al. Professional stereotypes among specialties and fields of work within the veterinary community. Vet Rec 2022;191(8):e1486.
7. Kinnison T, May SA. Veterinary career ambitions correlate with gender and past experience, with current experience influencing curricular perspectives. Vet Rec 2013;172(12):313.
8. Nelson LL, Friedli J, Hauptman J, et al. Evaluation of clinical grading and senior award receipt. Calgary, Alberta, Canada: Veterinary Educator Collaborative; 2016.
9. Sitkin NA, Pachankis JE. Specialty Choice Among Sexual and Gender Minorities in Medicine: The Role of Specialty Prestige, Perceived Inclusion, and Medical School Climate. LGBT Health 2016;3(6):451–60.
10. Gloria AM, Hird JS. Influences of Ethnic and Nonethnic Variables on the Career Decision-Making Self-Efficacy of College Students. Career Dev Q 2011;48(2): 157–74.
11. McGinn KL, Milkman KL. Looking up and looking out: Career mobility effects of demographic similarity among professionals. Organ Sci 2013;24(4):1041–60.
12. Banerjee R, Reitz JG, Oreopoulos P. Do large employers treat racial minorities more fairly? An analysis of Canadian field experiment data. University of Toronto Press Journals 2018;44(1):1–12.
13. Quillian L, Pager D, Hexel O, et al. Meta-analysis of field experiments shows no change in racial discrimination in hiring over time. Proc Natl Acad Sci U S A 2017. https://doi.org/10.1073/pnas.1706255114.
14. Poon SC, Nellans K, Gorroochurn P, et al. Race, But Not Gender, Is Associated With Admissions Into Orthopaedic Residency Programs. Clin Orthop Relat Res 2022;480(8):1441–9.
15. Wong RL, Sullivan MC, Yeo HL, et al. Race and surgical residency: results from a national survey of 4339 US general surgery residents. Ann Surg 2013;257(4): 782–7.
16. Byrne D. An Overview (and Underview) of Research and Theory within the Attraction Paradigm. J Soc Pers Relat 1997;14(3):291–431.
17. Hu C, Thomas KM, Lance CE. Intentions to initiate mentoring relationships: understanding the impact of race, proactivity, feelings of deprivation, and relationship roles. J Soc Psychol 2008;148(6):727–44.
18. Draper WR, Reid CA, McMahon BT. Workplace Discrimination and the Perception of Disability. Rehabil Counsel Bull 2011;55(1):29–37.
19. Loomans JBA, Van Weeren-Bitterling MS, Van Weeren PR, et al. Occupational disability and job satisfaction in the equine veterinary profession: How sustainable is this 'tough job'in a changing world? Equine Vet Educ 2008;20(11): 597–607.
20. Smits F, Houdmont J, Hill B, et al. Mental wellbeing and psychosocial working conditions of autistic veterinary surgeons in the UK. Vet Rec 2023;193(8):e3311.

21. Carr EW, Reece A, Kellerman GR, et al. The value of belonging at work. Harv Bus Rev 2019. Available at: https://hbr.org/2019/12/the-value-of-belonging-at-work.
22. Witte TK, Kramper S, Carmichael KP, et al. A survey of negative mental health outcomes, workplace and school climate, and identity disclosure for lesbian, gay, bisexual, transgender, queer, questioning, and asexual veterinary professionals and students in the United States and United Kingdom. J Am Vet Med Assoc 2020;257(4):417–31.
23. Summers OS, Medcalf R, Hubbard KA, et al. A cross-sectional study examining perceptions of discriminatory behaviors experienced and witnessed by veterinary students undertaking clinical extra-mural studies. Front Vet Sci 2023;10: 940836.
24. Freestone K, Remnant J, Gummery E. Gender discrimination of veterinary students and its impact on career aspiration: A mixed methods approach. Vet Rec Open 2022;9(1):e47.
25. Chung GH, Armitage-Chan E. Student Experience and Ethnic Diversity: The Experiences of Underrepresented Minority Students at a Veterinary University in the United Kingdom. J Vet Med Educ 2022;49(3):363–71.
26. Association AVM. AVMA 2023 Economic state of the profession. 2023.
27. Neill CL, Kakpo AT, Mack R. The role of experience, specialty certification, and practice ownership in the gender wage gap for veterinarians in the United States. J Am Vet Med Assoc 2021;258(6):591–600.
28. Field E, Krivkovich A, Kugele S, et al. Women in the workplace 2023. 2023. Available at: https://www.mckinsey.com/featured-insights/diversity-and-inclusion/women-in-the-workplace?utm_source=customer.io#/.
29. FitzGerald C, Hurst S. Implicit bias in healthcare professionals: a systematic review. BMC Med Ethics 2017;18(1):19.
30. Sabin JA, Greenwald AG. The influence of implicit bias on treatment recommendations for 4 common pediatric conditions: pain, urinary tract infection, attention deficit hyperactivity disorder, and asthma. Am J Public Health 2012;102(5): 988–95.
31. Schut RA. Racial disparities in provider-patient communication of incidental medical findings. Soc Sci Med 2021;277:113901.
32. Shen MJ, Peterson EB, Costas-Muñiz R, et al. The Effects of Race and Racial Concordance on Patient-Physician Communication: A Systematic Review of the Literature. J Racial Ethn Health Disparities 2018;5(1):117–40.
33. Cron WL, Slocum JV, Goodnight DB, et al. Executive summary of the Brakke management and behavior study. J Am Vet Med Assoc 2000;217(3):332–8.
34. Hoffman CL, Spencer TG, Makolinski KV. Assessing the Impact of a Virtual Shelter Medicine Rotation on Veterinary Students' Knowledge, Skills, and Attitudes Regarding Access to Veterinary Care. Front Vet Sci 2021;8:783233.
35. Perret J, Bateman S, Johns O, et al. Student Veterinarian Perceptions of Community-Based Primary Care Veterinary Clinics in Indigenous Communities in Southern Ontario, Canada. J Vet Med Educ 2023;e20220001. https://doi.org/10.3138/jvme-2022-0001.
36. Sukhera J, Watling CJ, Gonzalez CM. Implicit Bias in Health Professions: From Recognition to Transformation. Acad Med 2020;95(5):717–23.
37. Vela MB, Erondu AI, Smith NA, et al. Eliminating Explicit and Implicit Biases in Health Care: Evidence and Research Needs. Annu Rev Public Health 2022;43: 477–501.
38. Pettigrew TF. Intergroup contact theory. Annu Rev Psychol 1998;49:65–85.

39. Zheng L. To make lasting progress on DEI, measure outcomes. Harv Bus Rev 2023. Available at: https://hbr.org/2023/01/to-make-lasting-progress-on-dei-measure-outcomes.
40. Muragishi GA, Aguilar L, Carr PB, et al. Microinclusions: Treating women as respected work partners increases a sense of fit in technology companies. J Pers Soc Psychol 2023. https://doi.org/10.1037/pspi0000430.
41.. Tan JY, Poitras Pratt Y, Danyluk P. First, do no harm': systematic program evaluation of an equine veterinary service-learning initiative with Indigenous communities in Canada. BMC Med Educ 2024;24(1):287.

The Need for Diverse Leadership in Veterinary Medicine

Stephen Niño Cital, RVT, SRA, RLAT, CVPP, VTS-LAM, (Research Anesthesia)[a,b]

KEYWORDS

- Leadership • Critical mass • Innovation • Meritocracy • Privilege

KEY POINTS

- Diverse leadership increases innovation.
- Diverse leadership increases revenue.
- Diverse leaders must be listened to.
- Tokenization is harmful and nonproductive.
- Recruiting diverse leaders is a commitment.

INTRODUCTION

The veterinary industry continues to struggle with diversity at all levels, from pharmaceutical sales representative, nursing staff, to associate veterinarians, to board rooms. Our clients, whether they are pet owners or other veterinary professionals, deserve to feel comfortable by having those that serve, treat, lead, or own reflect our ever-diversifying world. In fact, people of color are expected to become the majority in the United States by 2042.[1]

In the veterinary industry, there is an intentional and long overdue paradigm shift occurring, in earnest, and as performance. Since around 2018, the veterinary industry has acknowledged its lack of racial diversity. Informative articles and statements on diversity issues are now common. Conscious inclusion by working toward diversity, equity, inclusion, and belonging (DEIB) efforts, such as incorporating DEIB talks at conferences is not unusual like it once was. The organization of various affinity and student groups is present and growing, and efforts in recruiting with diversity in mind is catching on. With these changes, one may think this is enough. It is not. Despite this shift, there are several notable blind spots and shortcomings. The paradigm shift mentioned is not reflected, as prevalent or rapidly, some would say at all, in leadership. The leadership in almost every professional sector often needs more diversity, from supervisors, to midlevel managers, to directors and executives, reflecting an outdated and exclusionary paradigm.

[a] Department of Neurobiology, Stanford University, 299 Campus Drive, Stanford, CA 94305, USA; [b] Remedy Veterinary Specialists, San Francisco, CA 94103, USA
E-mail address: matacital@gmail.com

Vet Clin Small Anim 54 (2024) 825–837
https://doi.org/10.1016/j.cvsm.2024.06.006 **vetsmall.theclinics.com**
0195-5616/24/

In this study, the focus will be on the importance of authentically including those who are Black, Indigenous, and other people of color (BIPOC)—those who are not White presenting—in leadership. This focus on the BIPOC community in veterinary leadership is not to diminish or ignore various other identities and their struggles, like sexual orientation, gender identity/presentation, disability, religion/ethno-religion, or place of birth, which often intersect with BIPOC people. Instead, studies that have looked at inclusionary work based on the various identities listed still find that leadership is racially homogenous. This study will also explore the ethical and business imperatives of fostering diverse leadership, its benefits, and the obstacles that need to be overcome to embrace the benefits of diverse leadership fully. Finally, this article is written candidly. It is not intended to make all readers comfortable. It is also not written to make readers feel defensive or angry, or meant to place blame or guilt. If one feels any of those feelings, one should sit with those feelings and ask why. Reflection on these emotions is the first step in truly becoming part of the solution rather than complicit in perpetuating structural racism and implicit biases. (More on implicit bias can be found in article titled, Jean-Yin Tan & Katherine Fogelberg's article, "Understanding Implicit Bias and Its Impact in Veterinary Medicine," in this issue.)

LEADERSHIP DEFINED

Leadership is a set of behaviors and/or social influence used to support individuals or a group in their collective direction to accomplish certain goals. *Professional leadership* is attributed to a person's title within an organization based on their defined position, seniority, or rank. Being a "leader" is not necessarily synonymous with professional leadership as an individual can have leadership qualities and influence without a title.[2,3]

The Uniqueness of Leadership in Veterinary Medicine

The veterinary industry offers a somewhat convoluted level of leadership in the clinical setting, given the structure of veterinary practice acts in North America. Unlike human medicine, where human nurses have their own practice acts, veterinary technicians, assistants, and other support staff fall under the legal supervision of the veterinarian on shift whether that veterinarian is defined as a "supervisor" on an organizational level or not. This introduces an important power dynamic for nonveterinarian staff that also warrants attention in discussions of diverse leadership.[4]

RACE AND ETHNICITY DEFINED

> *Race is a socially constructed system of categorizing human beings based on physically observable features, such as skin color, hair color, eye color, facial features, body types, and/or ancestry. Although race has been used to define people for centuries, there is no genetic basis for the classification…[**Table 1**]*
>
> *The term, ethnicity, refers to a group of people who share a common cultural back- ground, such as heritage, culture, ancestry, language, dialect, history, identity, or geographic origin. Members of the same ethnic group may come from the same country or live in the same area. For example, people who identify their origin as Hispanic, Latino, or Spanish may be of any race.*
>
> *—Odunayo & Ng, (2021) in Valuing Diversity in the Team, Veterinary Clinics of North America: Small Animal Practice*[5,6]

In March 2024, the Office of Information and Regulatory Affairs, Office of Management and Budget, and Executive Office of the President updated the racial and ethnicity categories that will be used by the government. This updated version delineates further groups that were once grouped together into separate answer categories and will improve US national demographic data.

THE WHITE RACE AND ITS PRIVILEGES

As seen in **Table 1**, the US government acknowledges and defines a White race. *White privilege*, often invisible to those holding it, refers to the unearned advantages enjoyed by White, or White passing individuals simply due to their skin color. The term has become heavily politicized with a negative connotation. However, this does not diminish or resolve the term as being based, in fact, as a systemic and embedded, measurable societal feature creating an uneven playing field. This privilege has been proven by numerous studies going back decades.[7]

Table 1
American Community Survey racial categories

US Federal Government's Race and Ethnicity Categories 1997	US Federal Government's Race and Ethnicity Categories 2024. (Adopted March 28, 2024) now Allowed to Mark All that Apply
Black or African American *A person having origins in any of the black racial groups of Africa*	Black or African American *African American, Jamaican, Haitian, Nigerian, Ethiopian, Somali, and so forth*
White *A person having origins in any of the original peoples of Europe, the Middle East, or North Africa*	White *English, German, Irish, Italian, Polish, Scottish, and so forth*
	Middle Eastern or North African *Lebanese, Iranian, Egyptian, Syrian, Iraqi, Israeli, and so forth*
American Indian or Alaska Native *A person having origins in any of the original peoples of North and South America (including Central America), and who maintains tribal affiliation or community attachment*	American Indian or Alaska Native *Navajo Nation, Blackfeet Tribe of the Blackfeet Indian Reservation of Montana, Native Village of Barrow Inupiat Traditional Government, Nome Eskimo Community, Aztec, Maya, and so forth*
Asian *A person having origins in any of the original peoples of the Far East, Southeast Asia, or the Indian subcontinent, including,* for example, *Cambodia, China, India, Japan, Korea, Malaysia, Pakistan, the Philippine Islands, Thailand, and Vietnam*	Asian *Chinese, Asian Indian, Filipino, Vietnamese, Korean, Japanese, and so forth*
Native Hawaiian or Other Pacific Islander *A person having origins in any of the original peoples of Hawaii, Guam, Samoa, or other Pacific Islands*	Native Hawaiian or Pacific Islander *Native Hawaiian, Samoan, Chamorro, Tongan, Fijian, Marshallese, and so forth*
**Ethnicity qualifier after checking a race category:* Hispanic or Latino *A person of Cuban, Mexican, Puerto Rican, Cuban, South or Central American, or other Spanish culture or origin, regardless of race*	Hispanic of Latino *Mexican, Puerto Rican, Salvadoran, Cuban, Dominican, Guatemalan, and so forth*

White privilege does not mean if one is White, one cannot suffer or face societal challenges. Many White people intersect with various minority and underrepresented groups, such as those who are Jewish, or challenges still faced by White women in historically male spaces. White privilege does not mean one does not have to work hard to accomplish the same goals as those who are not White. In North America and beyond, White privilege was built through centuries of colonization, enslavement, segregation, apartheid, scapegoating, and the deeply engrained implicit biases people developed against BIPOC communities, whether those biases are conscious or unconscious.[8] White privilege is best illustrated with a simple "yes or no" question asked to a White audience.

"Would you trade places with a Black person in today's society?"

Jane Elliot, a White woman who is internationally recognized as an educator on diversity, poses this same question in a slightly different way, *"I want every White person in this room who would be happy to be treated as this society in general treats our citizens, our Black citizens, if you, as a White person, would be happy to receive the same treatment that our Black citizens do in this society, please stand."*

The typical response is no answer or "no." Jane's response to this reaction is notable.

"That says very plainly that you know what's happening and you don't want it for you. I want to know why you're so willing to accept it or allow it to happen for others?"[9] (For more on being White in veterinary medicine, please see in the article, Amber Labelle's article, "What Does it Mean to Be White in Veterinary Medicine?," in this issue.)

Further solidifying White privilege as a legitimate concept is also seen in a different form: colorism within BIPOC communities.[10] The perceived benefits of White privilege has creeped into BIPOC communities over the centuries in the form of colorism, where lighter skin tones, or other physical traits such as the texture and color of one's hair, eye color or shape, anatomic features such as lip size and the shape of one's nose that are more European or White presenting are seen as desirable by certain BIPOC individuals and communities. White features are perceived to offer a person of color better opportunities in society or an easier time in assimilating (acting White).[11,12] It is also not uncommon to this day that people of color may personally want or encourage their children to procreate with a White person for its perceived benefits.

When your skin is seen as a weapon, you are never unarmed

—Regina Jackson

Manifestations of White privilege can be subtle or blatant. Examples include[13,14]

- Presuming one's safety and belonging in public spaces where non-White individuals may face suspicion or harassment.
- Benefitting from positive media portrayals and cultural narratives centered around whiteness, particularly those with power or perceived power.
- Having access to opportunities and resources historically denied to non-White communities due to discriminatory policies and practices.
- Navigating institutions (education, health care, and so forth) without encountering assumptions or microaggressions based on race.

WHY DIVERSITY IN LEADERSHIP MATTERS

Enhanced Innovation and Problem-solving

Businesses are always looking to boost innovation, keep or hire top talent, increase services, and, of course, increase revenue. With these common goals adopted throughout various industries, recommendations abound on how to achieve any or all of the points listed, from suggestions of hiring a Chief Innovation Officer to a magical "culture change" with little guidance on how to effectively achieve the change to hiring people from outside the classic pool of candidates in hopes of finding that one person(s) that can lead a new and successful charge.

Success with any of the aforementioned goals might come faster and more sustainably from another area not typically associated with improved business outcomes and diverse leadership teams. In 2017, Boston Consulting Group surveyed over 1600 companies in 8 countries across a number of industries and company sizes. This was a follow-up from a previous study where the researchers assessed various diversity paradigms to gauge the level of innovation based on total revenues over the last 3 years. One of the biggest conclusions identified was innovation (and revenues) increased in correlation to more diverse leadership. Companies that reported "average (nondiverse)" leadership fell 19 percentage points behind companies that reported above-average diverse leadership teams, with a 26% to 45% average innovation revenue increase reported.[15] A McKinsey study revealed that companies with ethnically diverse executive teams reaching "critical mass" were 33% more likely to outperform on profitability compared to less diverse executive teams. Diversity in leadership nurtures a more vibrant culture of originality, where different viewpoints are valued and encouraged, leading to more creative solutions.[16]

Critical Mass

One of the crucial factors in understanding how and when diverse leadership affects performance is the relative amount or proportion of diversity within a given group, from leadership to staff. This is because it is often the minority, whether in terms of gender, race, or other underrepresented identities, given their smaller voting share or cultural impact on the business, is hampered by representation alone in making meaningful influence on management decisions that could positively change overall business goals and even the conditions for the majority.[17] In other words, the number of people in a group who are outside of the majority demographic, with emphasis on gender and race, matters in terms of how and when diversity leads to negative, neutral, or positive results. However, reaching meaningful representation often comes with spoken and unspoken hurdles. Blalock, in 1967, argued that while minority groups can make gains, the majority group members lose something in return. This is also known as "zero-sum" thinking. This is because the majority group saw the minority group's size, mainly as more representation occurs, as a threat to their established positions and status quo. This is despite no real loss by anyone other than the visual representation and makeup of organizations sparking fear of the "other." This is more plainly an example of insidious structural racism and prejudice. In contrast, Kanter (1977) argued that both the minority and majority benefit from the resources the minority group members bring to the organization. However, these benefits only happen when there are enough minority group members to overcome the problems of tokenism.[18]

> ***"Token(s)"*** *is a term used to describe a person from a marginalized group that is amid the majority group that is generally more homogenous. The token usually has little impact on the group and can be used as "evidence" of inclusion.*

Additionally, it is not uncommon to have the majority group minimize or persuade the person from a marginalized group to fall in line with the majority group, cementing them as a *token* rather than a contributing voice. Other disingenuous efforts of inclusion involve prioritizing people from marginalized groups that align with the majority group's positions and perspectives, with that person from a historically marginalized group bucking the overall collective positions and opinions of the marginalized group they represent. While it is fair to say that people, no matter where they come from, are not a monolith, this intentional practice still occurs and is injurious. Malcom X is attributed to saying, "They will pay one of us, to kill one of us, just to say it was one of us."

Critical mass remains paramount regardless. As more and more people from different racial groups are added to a homogenous group, confines start to fade away. The minority votes and voices start to have more influence, which eventually improves equity and tips the traditional, less diverse leadership paradigm. What is critical mass as reflected by diversity in leadership? This is still contested given the nuances of the intersectionality of people in general and is hard to measure numerically. However, general percentages range from 20% to 35%. Simply reaching critical mass is important for understanding how and when diversity effects performance.[15,19,20]

Individuals that fall outside of the majority often experience some of the following[5]:

- Feeling the pressure to conform and make fewer mistakes
- Feeling more visible and on display
- Trying to become socially invisible so as not to stand out
- Finding it harder to gain credibility
- Being more isolated and underrespected
- Being more likely to be excluded from informal peer networks
- Having fewer opportunities to be sponsored
- Facing misperceptions about their identity and role in the organization
- Being more likely to be stereotyped
- Facing more personal stress
- Feeling like they did not earn their place (imposter syndrome) and were hired to check boxes as a token (ie, organizations hiring a racial or gender underrepresented individual to fulfill institutional hiring guidelines)
- Feeling underemployed and/or overused by departments or institutions
- Having their authority challenged by students and/or employees
- Having minimal guidance and mentoring toward promotion, tenure, and reappointment
- Dealing with colleagues who either ignore them or make racist comments about aspects, such as appearance or accent
- Disparagement of scholarly activity due to a focus on racial or ethnic issues

Deeper Client Understanding and Engagement

Understanding diverse customer segments is crucial for sustainable growth in today's globalized marketplace. When asking numerous BIPOC individuals for this study, Amber Labelle's article, "What Does it Mean to Be White in Veterinary Medicine?," in this issue, the responses often came back to the dynamics of the veterinarian as the leader in the context of client and staff engagement. BIPOC leaders naturally bring with them unique insights into different cultural nuances, consumer behaviors, and unmet needs within diverse communities. This allows companies to better tailor their products, services, and marketing strategies to reach a wider audience, resonate with previously underserved demographics, and ultimately drive customer and staff loyalty.

Diverse staff, including leadership, fosters cultural competency. Cultural competency is essential to understand as many people often do not appreciate that diversity is not only about having people that physically look or identify differently but also about the cultural differences and aspects that come along with authentic inclusion. Within veterinary medicine, this is an imperative as different cultural practices often intersect with various races that can impact the care of animals and approaches to dealing with staff and clients. Authentic cultural competency within leadership embraces new perspectives on traditionally Western or Eurocentric business and medical care practices.[21]

Cultural competency allows for a whole new demographic to feel comfortable and included whether that is for employment recruitment or clients. The rewards span from not only client and staff satisfaction and feelings of belonging or safety but also financial gain by including those previously ignored or underserved clients who feel accommodated in a practice. This also broadens the spectrum of care in veterinary medicine.[22,23]

In North America and many other parts of the world, we are still faced with generations of living people who were intentionally held back from certain professions or spaces because of blatant and structural racism. At the very least, because we live with generations that were limited or unsafe in certain places because of their race, it makes visible representation even more critical. Homogeneous leadership can lead to policies and practices that perpetuate discrimination and disadvantage marginalized communities.

Stronger Employer Branding and Talent Acquisition

Companies with diverse leadership teams project a more inclusive image, attracting top talent from diverse backgrounds who identify with and are inspired by leadership that looks like them. This not only broadens the talent pool but also fosters a more engaged and collaborative workforce, further fueling innovation and productivity. A Glassdoor study found that diversity in leadership increases a company's attractiveness to job seekers by 80%.[24]

Recruitment

Generation Z (people born after 2001) is on track to be one of the most educated and racially diverse generations yet in North America. A 2018 Pew Research Center study found Gen Z, like millennials (born 1981–2000), are more socially conscious than previous generations, with Gen Z having less tolerance and interest in working for employers that do not appear diversified racially and based on gender. Millennials and Gen Z customers also focus more attention on companies with diverse staff/leadership and will go out of their way to support companies that are more inclusive. Data from McKinsey & Co. found that the overall sentiment on diversity efforts was positive at 52% but also noticed how poorly those marginalized groups are included.[16]

How Recruitment and Hiring Practices Fail Black, Indigenous, and Other People of Color Individuals

Despite growing awareness of the importance of diversity in leadership, (BIPOC) individuals remain significantly underrepresented in leadership positions. One contributing factor is systemic failures within recruitment and hiring practices that create an uneven playing field.

Most commonly, we see failed hiring practices, especially for leadership roles, based on a number of areas that may not always be conscious[25,26]:

Unconscious bias

Implicit biases held by recruiters and hiring managers can influence decision-making, leading to the undervaluing of BIPOC candidates' qualifications and experiences. This bias can manifest in subtle ways, from focusing on perceived weaknesses to overlooking cultural nuances in resumes and interviews. Unconscious biases can be exacerbated by differences in presentation, such as hair styles, cultural garb, and jewelry. (See study, Jean-Yin Tan & Katherine Fogelberg's article, "Understanding Implicit Bias and Its Impact in Veterinary Medicine," in this issue.)

- *Homophily bias:* The tendency to favor candidates who share similar backgrounds can lead to hiring teams unconsciously perpetuating existing homogeneity. This can create a vicious cycle where diverse talent is consistently overlooked.
- *Lack of cultural competency:* Recruiters and hiring managers may lack the skills and awareness to effectively recognize and value the diverse experiences and perspectives of BIPOC candidates. This can lead to misinterpretations of resumes, awkward interview interactions, and an overall unwelcoming environment.
- *Standardized interviews:* Structured interviews can favor candidates who excel in traditional formats, potentially disadvantaging BIPOC candidates with different communication styles or cultural backgrounds. People who speak with an accent are at an increased risk of a negative bias. Additionally, the lack of diverse interview panels can further perpetuate unconscious bias.
- *Unconscious algorithmic bias:* Even seemingly objective algorithms used in resume screening can perpetuate bias by being trained on skewed data sets. This can lead to qualified BIPOC candidates being automatically filtered out before human reviewers even see their applications.

Mentorship

If one were to look at the 2023 to 2024 American Veterinary Medical Association's (AVMA) executive team and Board of Directors, the diversity scorecard would be a losing one. Based on the headshots of the leaders alone, the AVMA leaders appear homogenous.[27] When professionals aspire to grow, they often find the best mentorship comes from someone who can relate to their lived experience, understands the challenges they may have gone through, and communicates in a similar way (verbally or nonverbally) to build personal connection. Not seeing a familiar face is discouraging and can even create a feeling of discomfort and isolation or a feeling that the position or space is not meant for them. Currently, all levels of veterinary medicine do not reflect North America's ever diversifying demographics leading to poorer mentorship for BIPOC community that can lead to professional advancement.[28]

Enhanced Brand Reputation and Social Impact

As briefly mentioned earlier, today's ever socially conscious consumer increasingly makes purchasing decisions based on a company's values and commitment to diversity and inclusion. Having BIPOC leaders demonstrates a company's dedication to these values, enhancing brand reputation and customer loyalty and attracting socially responsible investors. A study by Cone Communications found that more than 80% of global consumers consider a company's social impact when making purchasing decisions.[29]

Improved Decision-making and Risk Management

Diversity in leadership fosters a culture of questioning assumptions and challenging the status quo, leading to more thorough analysis and well-rounded decision-making. This reduces the risk of groupthink and ensures that diverse perspectives are considered, mitigating potential blind spots, and improving risk management. A study by Deloitte found that diverse leadership teams are 87% more likely to consider multiple perspectives before making important decisions.[30] An authentically diverse leadership team will also help decrease potential lawsuits based on discrimination claims.[19]

Groupthink is a psychological phenomenon that occurs within a group of people when the desire for harmony or conformity in the group results in an irrational or dysfunctional decision-making outcome. Group members try to minimize conflict and reach a consensus decision without critical evaluation of alternative viewpoints.

The Meritocracy Myth

Proponents of meritocracy alone argue that individuals should be rewarded based on their qualifications and achievements, regardless of background or identity. This "level playing field" seems inherently fair, promoting individual effort and rewarding talent.

However, one must not ignore the historical and systemic disadvantages that created an uneven playing field for marginalized groups. Meritocracy alone ignores these realities, perpetuating existing inequalities and masking discriminatory practices.[31] If meritocracy alone was a viable and fair system, we would not still be living in the age of "firsts." In the last 20 years alone, the low end of time considered a "generation," we have seen the first Black president, the first Black/South Asian woman vice president, the first Latina Supreme Court Justice, the first openly gay and Latino AVMA president, and so forth.

When companies or organizations adopt the "We can't find 'qualified' candidates" line, we also must ask ourselves, does a long history of structural racism have anything to do with it? Do the barriers of the past and present contribute to the "lack" of talent? Or are companies and organizations not looking hard enough or with honest intentions? Conversely, a person being BIPOC should be looked at as an additional qualifier particularly when studies show the business advantages of maintaining diverse leadership.[32,33]

Black, Indigenous, and Other People of Color and Other Minority Groups Interpersonal Accountability

Personal accountability is critical for the growth and success of anyone. BIPOC individuals are also not immune from actively learning about other communities and cultures. People from marginalized groups may appear to have a "pass" because they are part of a marginalized group. This is not true, fair, or appropriate. A recent example in veterinary medicine involved 2 leaders who are part of 2 different minority groups who signed off on, and participated in dressing up in costumes that fall into blatantly harmful stereotypes about a specific culture neither leader is a part of as an activity during a conference they organized. They were called-in about the pictures of them in the costumes and were removed from their social media accounts. How can BIPOC or other minority communities expect anyone to do better when harmful actions are perpetuated by minority community members themselves? DEIB training is not only for our White colleagues but also for everyone.

> *Calling in is an invitation to a one-on-one or small group conversation to bring attention to an individual or group's harmful words or behavior, including bias, prejudice, microaggressions, and discrimination.*[34]

Another harmful practice commonly practiced by BIPOC communities is changing individual behaviors, mannerisms, hairstyles, dress and even dialect, code switching, to appease White colleagues. This only further perpetuates that BIPOC expression is "less than." Fitting in is not equality, it is compromise and conforming.

Broadly, code-switching involves adjusting one's style of speech, appearance, behavior, and expression in ways that will optimize the comfort of others in exchange for fair treatment, quality service, and employment opportunities.[35]

Since DEIB efforts started, there have been those actively and aggressively trying to dismantle DEIB work. An alarming and growing number of attempts are successful. What is particularly jarring is the narrative claims that DEIB is "divisive" and creates "division." Several states in the United States have passed laws meant to diminish, ban, and rewrite the history of BIPOC people.[36,37] Books meant to encourage BIPOC children to reach for more are being banned, like *Little Leaders, Bold Women in Black History* by Vachti Harrison, with the excuse that they make White children feel uncomfortable. Is highlighting the positive contributions of BIPOC people really that scary when all children in North America have been educated on hundreds of years of White men's successes and conquests?[38] This flip is based in White supremacy and discomfort in discussions about race despite a lack of evidence to show any true harm toward people who are considered White—feelings of discomfort aside.[39–41]

Even more disastrous is the in-fighting of marginalized communities and attempts to completely dismantle DEIB efforts since the October 7, 2023 attack in Israel.[42–44] As an example, in early 2024, the American Academy of Dermatology received a member-led resolution to dismantle the academy's DEIB initiatives completely. The resolution was based on other DEIB group and organizations' perceived failures, not the academy's, as stated in a poorly referenced resolution.

"DEI, in its current form, is believed to contribute to a decrease in the ability to provide unbiased and equal medical care for everyone, as it is seen to foster division rather than unity; and WHEREAS, since October 7th, there have been instances where the DEI movement has been perceived as being filled with antisemitism, weaponizing the concept against Jews by labeling them as "oppressors" and allegedly justifying extreme hate speech and violence; and WHEREAS, Judaism is a religion, culture, and race that does not inherently fit within the DEI framework of oppressor and oppressed classes, and many Jews do not fit within the preconceived racial categories, challenging the binary system DEI promotes; and WHEREAS, the world's complexity cannot be adequately addressed by a simplistic dichotomous system, and every patient should be treated equally without viewing them through the lens of oppressor or oppressed; and WHEREAS, many professionals have dedicated their careers to advocating for and supporting disadvantaged communities, and the current DEI system, which is perceived to contain antisemitic elements, is seen as inconsistent with these values; and WHEREAS, DEI, while initially well-intentioned, is now believed to hinder rather than help the diversity in our specialty and the broader healthcare field, and to obstruct efforts to address and improve racism within our systems"

What is alarming about this resolution and the statements made by predominately White or White presenting Jewish academy members is the effort to totally dismantle an initiative that they see as oppressive for one part of a person's identity. To claim it "hinders" rather than helps diversity or that the efforts are unfairly serving one marginalized group over another is false and an example of privilege based solely on a less visible part of an identity that BIPOC, non-White presenting people do not have. Often lost in these actions or uncomfortable conversations is tangible proof or evidence of harm, instead leaning on personal opinions or perceptions. When predominately White people present resolutions like this, it is also not uncommon that their feelings and assumptions, without tangible proof, often outweigh and take precedence over the measurable harm and struggles based on structural hurdles encountered by BIPOC people. Whereas dismantling an entire DEIB effort instead of finding solutions while still maintaining the privilege of being part of, or passing, in the dominant group is inherently oppressive and racist.[43] Dismantling DEIB efforts will embolden those who seek to harm BIPOC people.[44,45] Minority communities must make it imperative to work together despite our shortcomings and differences.[46]

Ignorance allied with power is the most ferocious enemy justice can have.
—James Baldwin

SUMMARY

Incorporating BIPOC individuals into leadership roles goes beyond just meeting diversity quotas. Leadership teams with members from a variety of backgrounds bring a rich mix of experiences, perspectives, and strategies to the table. While promoting DEIB for moral reasons is essential, the benefits of hiring and recruiting BIPOC individuals for leadership go beyond ethics. Studies and observations in the marketplace indicate a strong connection between team diversity, and several positive outcomes. This approach not only improves how a business operates but also significantly increases profits, decreases staff turnover, and attracts the top talent.

DISCLOSURE

The author has no disclosures.

REFERENCES

1. Daniel A. Creating a Path to Diversity in the Veterinary Profession. Today's Veterinary Practice. 2021. Available at: https://www.researchgate.net/profile/Annie-Daniel/publication/351346762_Creating_a_Path_to_Diversity_in_the_Veterinary_Profession/links/6092882ca6fdccaebd096dd6/Creating-a-Path-to-Diversity-in-the-Veterinary-Profession.pdf. [Accessed 2 February 2024].
2. Prentice WCH. Understanding Leadership. Harv Bus Rev 2004. Available at: https://hbr.org/2004/01/understanding-leadership.
3. McKinsey. What Is leadership: a Definition and Way Forward | McKinsey. Available at: www.mckinsey.com. [Accessed 17 August 2022] https://www.mckinsey.com/featured-insights/mckinsey-explainers/what-is-leadership.
4. RESOLUTION #10-2023 Regular. Annual Session SAFEGUARDING CARE for ANIMALS with VETERINARIAN-LED TEAMS. Available at: https://www.avma.org/sites/default/files/2023-06/2023S_Resolution10-Safeguarding.pdf. [Accessed 24 February 2024].
5. Odunayo & Ng. Valuing diversity in the team. Vet Clin Small Anim Pract 2021; 51(5):1009–40.
6. Census.gov. 2023. Available at: https://www.census.gov/quickfacts/fact/note/US/RHI625222.
7. Leonardo Z. The Color of Supremacy: Beyond the discourse of "white privilege.". Educ Philos Theor 2004;36(2):137–52.
8. Wildman SM. The Persistence of White Privilege. Wash Univ J Law Pol 2005;18:245–66.
9. A Powerful Lesson in Discrimination. kottke.org. Available at: https://kottke.org/20/06/a-powerful-lesson-in-discrimination. [Accessed 24 February 2024].
10. Branigan AR, Wildeman C, Freese J, et al. Complicating Colorism: Race, Skin Color, and the Likelihood of Arrest. Socius: Sociological Research for a Dynamic World 2017;3. 237802311772561.

11. Nguyen M. Colorism: The psychological effects of skin color discrimination among Ethnic/Racial minority women. [Order No. 28965450]. Adler Univeristy ProQuest Dissertations & Thesis; 2022.
12. Burton LM, Bonilla-Silva E, Ray V, et al. Critical Race Theories, Colorism, and the Decade's Research on Families of Color. J Marriage Fam 2010;72(3):440–59.
13. Dei GJS, Karumanchery LL, Karumanchery-Luik N. White Power, White Privilege. Counterpoints 2004;244:81–99 [date you accessed the site]. Available at: http://www.jstor.org/stable/42979560.
14. Grindstaff K, Mascarenhas M. "No One Wants to Believe It": Manifestations of White Privilege in a STEM-Focused College. Multicult Perspect 2019;21(2):102.
15. Lorenzo R, Voigt N, Tsusaka M, et al. How diverse leadership teams boost innovation. 2018. Available at: http://boston-consulting-group-brightspot.s3.amazonaws.com/img-src/BCG-How-Diverse-Leadership-Teams-Boost-Innovation-Jan-2018_tcm9-207935.pdf.
16. How diversity, equity, and inclusion (DE&I) matter | McKinsey. Available at: www.mckinsey.com https://www.mckinsey.com/featured-insights/diversity-and-inclusion/diversity-wins-how-inclusion-matters#/.
17. Lefley F, Janeček V. Board gender diversity, quotas and critical mass theory. Corp Commun Int J 2023. https://doi.org/10.1108/ccij-01-2023-0010. Published online April 13.
18. Fredette C, Sessler Bernstein R. Ethno-racial Diversity on Nonprofit Boards: A Critical Mass Perspective. Nonprofit Voluntary Sect Q 2019;48(5):931–52.
19. Miksch KL. Legal Issues in Developmental Education: Affirmative Action, Race, and Critical Mass. Res Teach Dev Educ 2003;20(1):69–76. Available at: http://www.jstor.org/stable/42802551.
20. Garces LM, Jayakumar UM. Dynamic Diversity. Educ Res 2014;43(3):115–24.
21. Paasche-Orlow M. The Ethics of Cultural Competence. Acad Med 2004;79(4):347–50.
22. Schilder AJ, Kennedy C, Goldstone IL, et al. "Being dealt with as a whole person." Care seeking and adherence: the benefits of culturally competent care. Soc Sci Med 2001;52(11):1643–59.
23. Betancourt JR, Green AR. Commentary: Linking Cultural Competence Training to Improved Health Outcomes: Perspectives From the Field. Acad Med 2010;85(4):583–5.
24. Glassdoor. Recruiting a Diverse Workforce | Glassdoor for Employers. US | Glassdoor for Employers 2021. Available at: https://www.glassdoor.com/employers/blog/diversity/.
25. Kessler J, Low C. Research: How Companies Committed to Diverse Hiring Still Fail. Harv Bus Rev 2021. Available at: https://hbr.org/2021/02/research-how-companies-committed-to-diverse-hiring-still-fail.
26. Newton L. Diversity and inclusion: how hiring practices are failing BIPOC workers. Sogolytics Blog; 2022. Available at: https://www.sogolytics.com/blog/how-hiring-practices-are-failing-bipoc-workers/. [Accessed 25 February 2024].
27. AVMA volunteer leaders. American veterinary medical association. Available at: www.avma.org. [Accessed 15 February 2024] https://www.avma.org/about/avma-volunteer-leaders.
28. Ofosu DH. Why Your Organization Needs a BIPOC Mentorship Program (Part 1). I/O Advisory Services Inc. 2021. Available at: https://ioadvisory.com/why-your-organization-needs-a-bipoc-mentorship-program/. [Accessed 15 February 2024].
29. MacCarthy L. New Report Reveals 86% of US Consumers Expect Companies to Act on Social, Environmental Issues. Sustainable Brands. 2017. Available at:

https://sustainablebrands.com/read/marketing-and-comms/new-report-reveals-86-of-us-consumers-expect-companies-to-act-on-social-environmental-issues.
30. Verschoor CC. Millennials' view of business ethics sinks sharply: A Deloitte survey finds that younger professionals are taking an increasingly negative view of businesses' motivations and ethics. Strat Finance 2018;100(2):20. Gale Academic OneFile. Accessed February 25, 2024.
31. Powell S, Arora-Jonsson S. The conundrums of formal and informal meritocracy: dealing with gender segregation in the academy. High Educ 2021. https://doi.org/10.1007/s10734-021-00719-2.
32. Anne Bell L, Funk MS. Racism, white supremacy and finding justice for all. Taylor & Francis Group: Routledge eBooks; 2022. p. 135–76. Published online June 27.
33. Barone RP, Mora F. Equity Is Not Equality: Prioritization, Preference and Privilege on the Neoliberal College Campus. About Campus 2023;28(5):62–7.
34. Calling in and Calling out Guide What Is Calling in and Calling Out?. Available at: https://edib.harvard.edu/files/dib/files/calling_in_and_calling_out_guide_v4.pdf.
35. McCluney C, Robotham K, Lee S, et al. The Costs of Code-Switching. Harv Bus Rev 2019. Available at: https://hbr.org/2019/11/the-costs-of-codeswitching.
36. Catherine T. DEI efforts are under siege. Here's what experts say is at stake. CNN; 2024. Available at: https://www.cnn.com/2024/01/07/us/dei-attacks-experts-warn-of-consequences-reaj/index.html.
37. Hinton A Jr, Shuler HD, Murray SA, et al. Climbing the mountain of adversity and removing barriers along the path. iScience 2023;27(1):108510. https://doi.org/10.1016/j.isci.2023.108510. Published 2023 Dec 19.
38. Banned Books 2022 – Little Leaders: Bold Women in Black History – Marshall Libraries. Available at: https://www.marshall.edu/library/bannedbooks/little-leaders/. [Accessed 26 February 2024].
39. Iyer A. Understanding advantaged groups' opposition to diversity, equity, and inclusion (DEI) policies: The role of perceived threat. Social and Personality Psychology Compass 2022;16(5). https://doi.org/10.1111/spc3.12666.
40. Zheng L. How to Effectively — and Legally — Use Racial Data for DEI. Harv Bus Rev 2023. Available at: https://hbr.org/2023/07/how-to-effectively-and-legally-use-racial-data-for-dei.
41. Watson L. Anti-DEI efforts are the latest attack on racial equity and free speech | ACLU. American Civil Liberties Union; 2024. Available at: https://www.aclu.org/news/free-speech/anti-dei-efforts-are-the-latest-attack-on-racial-equity-and-free-speech.
42. Lederman J. Why Jews must dismantle diversity, equity, and inclusion (DEI). Jewish Journal; 2024. Available at: https://jewishjournal.org/2024/01/31/why-jews-must-dismantle-diversity-equity-and-inclusion-dei/. [Accessed 25 February 2024].
43. Glaude E. DEI is not the monster here. TIME; 2023. Available at: https://time.com/6458406/dei-campus-speech/. [Accessed 26 February 2024].
44. Emerson J. The anti-DEI movement has gone from fringe to mainstream. Here's what that means for corporate America. Fortune. Available at: https://fortune.com/2024/01/04/anti-dei-movement-fringe-mainstream-corporate-america-diversity-equity-inclusion-meaning-joelle-emerson/.
45. Levin S. DEI programs can harm Jews — but they don't have to. JIMENA 2023. Available at: https://www.jimena.org/dei-programs-can-harm-jews-but-they-dont-have-to/. [Accessed 25 February 2024].
46. Cohen H. Jewish communal leaders still committed to DEI framework, despite widespread criticism. Jewish Insider; 2023. Available at: https://jewishinsider.com/2023/12/diversity-equity-and-inclusion-american-jewish-committee-anti-defamation-league/. [Accessed 25 February 2024].

What Does It Mean to Be White in Veterinary Medicine?

Amber Labelle, DVM, MS*

KEYWORDS

• Race • Social construct • Identity • White supremacy • Intersectionality

KEY POINTS

- Race is a human-invented system of categorization using skin color as a proxy for intelligence. It has no biologic basis.
- The history of veterinary medicine has helped shape veterinary medicine into the whitest profession in the United States.
- Race is not real, but racism is.
- You do not have to feel guilty for the things your ancestors did; you do have to work to make things better in the future.

INTRODUCTION

There's often this hesitation of: I'm not perfect, therefore, I shouldn't. And so it's sort of become this chant to myself that

I don't have to be perfect to do good.

— *'Cúagilákv (Jess Housty), Haíłzaqv (Heiltsuk) Nation.*[1]

As veterinary practitioners, there are high expectations for the quality of our work. Ligatures should not slip, injections should be given into the correct vessel, and drugs should be dosed accurately. The consequences of mistakes can be devastating, if not fatal, for the creatures whose care is entrusted to us. Living with the pressure to sustain excellence is not only exhausting, but can lead to "perfection creep", wherein we start to view actions or tasks as requiring perfection when they actually do not.[2]

One place white veterinary professionals often feel we must be perfect is in the discussion of race. Is our fear of making mistakes in this realm the same as our fear of making mistakes in the operating room? While we know all too well the fatal,

Bright Light Veterinary Eye Care, Ottawa, Ontario, Canada
* 1445 Merivale Road #102, Nepean, ON, K2E 5N9, Canada.
E-mail address: hello@brightlightvet.ca
Twitter: @brightlightvet (A.L.)

Vet Clin Small Anim 54 (2024) 839–848
https://doi.org/10.1016/j.cvsm.2024.06.007 vetsmall.theclinics.com
0195-5616/24/

hemorrhagic consequences of a slipped ligature, why do we project the fear of that consequence onto our discussions of race and identity? Are we afraid of doing harm to our BIPOC (Black, Indigenous, and People of Color) colleagues? Do we fear imperfection and doing or saying the wrong thing? Do we worry we will be judged solely on our mistakes?

Setting perfectionism aside and embracing our mistakes gives us the space to learn and the courage to grow, especially in discussions and actions about race.[3] Neither can we allow our fear of mistakes to dominate our discussions of race and identity, nor can we allow perfectionism to prevent us from taking action: the reality of racism is simply too grave. This article is written by me, a white veterinarian, for my fellow white veterinarians. The purpose of this article is to help us think more deeply about our white racial identity, how we relate to the world, and how to be a force for good in veterinary medicine.

WHAT IS RACE?

You may have heard the phrase "race is a social construct". What this means is: race is a story made up by humans to put other humans in categories based on the color of their skin. It has no biologic basis.[4]

To be clear: skin color is real. Skin color is a reflection of the amount of melanin in the dermis. Skin color is both heritable and environmental. Three factors influence skin color: the amount of melanin in the skin, your ancestors, and your exposure to ultraviolet (UV) light.[5] Skin color can change with UV light exposure and with age. While we use the phrases "white" and "Black" to describe skin color, all skin is different shades of brown, from very light to very dark.[5]

Race "science" emerged in the 1700s as early scientists worked to classify the natural world. Swedish scientist Carl Linnaeus, who we all studied in our undergraduate biology classes, classified humans into 4 groups and assigned to them characteristics based on skin color.[6] Working initially with measurements of skulls, German scientist Johann Blumenbach declared the "Caucasian" race, named for the nearby Caucasus Mountains, to be the superior race.[7] Skull measurements of people of different skin colors were used as a proxy for intelligence. Race "science" persisted through several centuries and was used as justification for the enslavement of Africans, the murder of Native Americans, and the domination of white Europeans over North America.[8] Race "science" has now been thoroughly discredited and widely rejected by scholars, clinicians, scientists, and social scientists.[9]

The phenotypic trait skin color as a distinguishing characteristic was arbitrarily selected. Early scientists could have selected eye color, height, ear shape, or toe length. Why was skin color selected? Perhaps because it was an easily observable characteristic.[4] Skin color cannot be used to sort humans into distinct groups because the human species is only 1 species. We cannot be divided into races or "breeds". Race is a made-up categorization that falsely sorts humans into different groups when in fact, we are all one human race.

Medical education is moving away from a "racial essentialism" view that ties specific diseases to racial categories toward the complete elimination of race-based medicine.[9] Earlier medical education associated some diseases, such as sickle cell anemia, with race. We now understand that the sickle cell trait is more prevalent in geographic regions where malaria is present rather than being inherently related to skin color.[10] Race-conscious medicine rejects the false idea that race is biologic and allows for awareness, reduction, and ultimately elimination of racial health disparities. Genetic researchers continue to update language and reporting standards on race, ethnicity, and ancestry.[11]

WHY HUMAN RACE AND CANINE BREED ARE NOT THE SAME?

Race is not real; humans are not biologically different based on their skin color alone.[6] Skin color is a phenotypic trait with a continuous spectrum of expression. Scholar and social worker Kay McChesney's 6 principles remind us that race has no biologic basis (**Box 1**).

As veterinarians, we may be asked how humans differ from the species we treat. How are canine breeds different from humans? Is "race" the same as "breed"?

No. Race is not the same as breed.[12]

Dog breeds differ in their genetic variation, with up to 27% of deoxyribonucleic acid (DNA) differing between breeds.[13] Genetics can be used to identify individual dogs of different breeds with 99% accuracy.[12] Humans genetic variation is only 2% to 3% of our DNA, with more variation being detected within geographically similar populations of humans than between humans of different skin colors.[12] Genetics cannot differentiate humans of different skin colors.[12] We can say with confidence, supported by the data, that there is only one human race, and neither there are breeds nor subspecies of humans.

RACE AND COLOR-BLINDNESS

Have you ever heard someone say "I treat all people equally; it doesn't matter if you are white or Black or purple or green, I don't see your color"? This is racial color-blindness.

In her book "The Sum of Us: What Racism Costs Everyone and How We Can Prosper Together", author Heather McGee writes:

> *When I was growing up in the 1980s, we were taught that the way to be a good person was to swear that race didn't matter, at least not anymore.*
>
> *We had all learned the lessons of the civil rights movement—that everybody is equal, and according to the morals of the sitcoms we watched after school (Diff'rent Strokes, Webster, Saved by the Bell), what was racist was pretending that people were any different from one another. Furthermore, the most un-racist people did not even see race at all; they were color blind.*
>
> *We now know that color blindness is a form of racial denial that took one of the aspirations of the civil rights movement—that individuals would one day "not be judged by the color of their skin but by the content of their character"—and*

Box 1
The 6 principles of race having no biologic basis from teaching diversity: The science you need to know to explain why race is not biologic[6]

1. People cannot be reliably divided into racial groups.
2. There are no relationships between traits that are used to categorize people into races (like skin color) and associated stereotypes.
3. Over time, geography and environment influence the genetic structures of human populations through natural selection.
4. There is more diversity within racial groups than between racial groups.
5. All people living today are descended from populations that originated in Africa.
6. All people living today are one biologic species.

stripped it from any consideration of power, hierarchy, or structure. The moral logic and social appeal of color blindness is clear, and many well-meaning people have embraced it. But when it is put into practice in a still-racist world, the result is more racism.[14]

The pervasiveness of this color-blind worldview has caused tremendous harm.[15] Instead of contributing to a veterinary profession where everyone is seen as equal, color-blindness erases unique differences between people and creates more inequality. Dr. Lisa Greenhill of the American Association of Veterinary Medical Colleges shares:

I am a richly melanated African American woman. Folks without vision issues who look at me and claim to not see my brown skin are not being truthful with me or themselves. Moreover, their unwillingness to see and acknowledge my race makes me wonder if these folks can see and acknowledge the racism I have experienced as a result of my race.[15]

Color-blind ideology also helps provide a cover story for the myth of race. If the prevailing logic is "I see all people as equal regardless of color", then there is no reason to learn about the reality of race, why race has no biologic basis and the impacts of racism on veterinary professionals.

WHY RACE MATTERS (EVEN THOUGH IT IS MADE UP)?

Understanding the fiction and ideas around race is important because they permeate our daily lives and are part of our identity.[16] While race is not real, racism is. The stories humans have invented and repeated about who we are and who others are have real impacts.[17] Racist ideas shape economic policy, educational policy, health policy, and housing policy.[14] The staggering wealth gap experienced by Black Americans is directly related to the effects of enslavement, housing policies that denied investment in Black neighborhoods, and predatory loan and banking practices.[14] The legacy of the inaccurate story humans invented about race means we are living with the consequences of repeating this false story for generations.

Race is broader than a Black and white binary. BIPOC veterinarians of non-white identities are underrepresented in veterinary medicine.[18] Experiences of racism and discrimination have been given more public visibility in recent years.[19,20] The bulk of the data presented here focuses on the experiences of Black Americans because the pervasive and pernicious nature of anti-Black racism dictates that we should explore its roots in order to rid our communities of its impacts.[17] Improving conditions for Black veterinarians means improving conditions for all veterinarians (**Fig. 1**).

Veterinary medicine was *the* whitest profession in the United States (US) until 2022, when we had to share the title with speech language pathologists.[21,22] This means veterinarians are disproportionately white compared to the US general population, ranging from 95% of the profession in 2014 to 90% in 2022. The lack of race-based data collection likely obscures a similar pattern in Canada.[23] How did we become the whitest profession?

THE (VERY WHITE) HISTORY OF VETERINARY MEDICINE

Veterinary medicine has existed for thousands of years. Humans and animals have had intimate relationships since time immemorial, and humans have been caretakers for as long as these relationships have existed.[24] The first contemporary Western veterinary school was founded in Lyon, France in 1761.[25] At the time, the major focus of

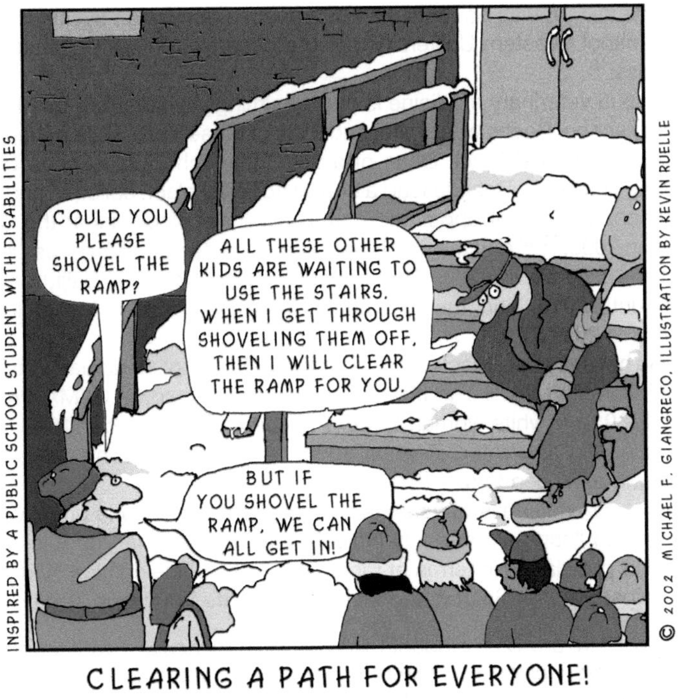

Fig. 1. Clearing a Path. "Clearing a Path" cartoon with permission from University of Vermont Center for Digital Initiatives and Absurdities and Realities of Special Education. The cartoon shows children attempting to enter school building. One of the school staff members is busy shoveling the snow-covered stairs. A disabled, wheelchair user child asks the staff member "Can you please shovel the ramp?" The staff member replies "All these other kids are waiting to use the stairs. When I get through shoveling them off, then I will clear the ramp for you." The original child replies "But if you shovel the ramp, we can all get in!" This cartoon shows how when we plan and execute with the needs of the people who are excluded, we meet everyone's needs more effectively and efficiently. When we center the needs of Black veterinarians in our planning, policies, and practices, veterinary medicine improves for everyone.

veterinary medicine was horses and livestock, with an urgent emphasis on herd health as a result of Rinderpest decimating European cattle herds. When the first private US (1852), public US (1879), and Canadian (1862) veterinary schools opened, much like the school in France, the classes consisted entirely of white men.[26] The first Black veterinarian in the US, Dr. Augustus Nathaniel Lushington, did not graduate until 1897, and the first Black female veterinarians in the US (Drs. Jane Hinton and and Alfreda Johnson Webb) did not graduate until 1949.[27] In the nearly 60 year interval between 1889 and 1948, only 70 Black veterinarians were graduated in the US and Canada.[28] For comparison, the American Veterinary Medical Association (AVMA) had approximately 13,000 members by 1948.[29]

Tuskegee University College of Veterinary Medicine was founded in 1945 "to provide an opportunity for an ethnic minority largely denied admission to the existing veterinary schools".[28] This mission was made necessary by the violent segregation that kept Black students from attending other veterinary schools.[30] Since its founding, Tuskegee has graduated more BIPOC veterinarians than any other veterinary school, and is the only veterinary school to consistently graduate classes that are less than 50%

BIPOC students.[28] It was not until the 2022 to 2023 admission cycle that another US veterinary school (Western University) selected nearly 50% BIPOC students for their entering class.[18]

Leadership in veterinary medicine is overwhelmingly white. Prior to 2018, 96.3% of all veterinary school Deans was white, and 91% of those were white men.[31] Dr Edward Evans became the first Black Dean of a veterinary school (Tuskegee University) in 1946, but the first Black Dean to lead a non-historically black colleges and universities veterinary school was not appointed until Dr Michael Blackwell at the University of Tennessee in 2000.[28,32] and the first Black woman to be appointed was Dr Ruby Perry at Tuskegee University in 2015. The first south Asian Dean (Dr Baljit Singh) was not appointed until 2016, and the first Latin Dean (Dr Carmen Fuentealba) was not appointed until 2017.[31]

There has never been a Black president of the AVMA nor Canadian Veterinary Medical Association (CVMA).[33] The first white woman to become CVMA President was elected in 1989, first white woman AVMA President was elected in 1996, and the first white woman was appointed Dean in 1998, all milestones achieved well ahead of BIPOC people of all genders.[29,31,34]

The persistent whiteness of veterinary medicine has not gone unnoticed. In 2004, observers noted "numbers strongly indicate that the veterinary profession does not reflect the US population in terms of race."[35] A 2003 article entitled "Veterinary Medicine: The Most Racially Segregated Field in Graduate Education Today" noted.

> *Combined, there are 1232 students enrolled at the schools of veterinary medicine at Oregon State University, Texas A&M University, the University of Minnesota, and Washington State University. Not one is [B]lack.*[36]

Black people comprised approximately 13% of the population in 2003, and Black students comprised 4% or less of veterinary school classes at every university but Tuskegee that year.[36] The author offers a comparison of the effects of segregationist Jim Crow laws on Black Americans entering veterinary medicine versus other professional fields such as medicine or banking:

> *By [1945], a vast majority of African Americans had moved off the farm and lived in the nation's cities. Most [B]lacks who remained on the farm were farm laborers who worked for whites. Generally, it was whites who owned the livestock that required the care of a veterinarian. Even for African Americans who owned farms, white practitioners of veterinary medicine seldom held any bias against the pets of farm animals of [B]lack people. Animals were animals and the race of their owners was not a major concern. As a result, there was not a demand for the development of a segregated class of [B]lack veterinarians. To be sure, if a [B]lack person were to enter the profession of veterinary medicine, he or she would have had slim pickings as the vast majority of whites would no more engage a [B]lack veterinarian than they would go to a [B]lack medical doctor or dentist.*[36]

These snapshots of the history of veterinary medicine help answer the question "Why is veterinary medicine so white?" Contemporary veterinary medicine was founded by and for white cisgender men, and it is partly through racist exclusion that veterinary medicine has remained so white.

IT MATTERS THAT YOU ACKNOWLEDGE YOU ARE WHITE

Who you are, racially, matters to your daily life. When you walk into the clinic to start your day, you bring your whole entire self to work with you. You cannot leave your skin color and other people's perception of you at the door! Every single person in your clinic, including you, has a racial identity. One of the pitfalls of the color-blind ideology that we discussed earlier is the central tendency to view white as "normal" or "baseline". This allows white people to view themselves neutrally while viewing others as having a racial identity.[37] This then allows white people to overlook the impact their own racial identity has on themselves and those around them.

White is not a neutral identity because while race is not real, racism in veterinary medicine is.

In a 2014 study, nearly 30% of BIPOC American veterinary students reported hearing racist comments in school frequently or very frequently.[38] In a 2022 study of Canadian veterinarians, 50% of BIPOC veterinarians report experiencing discrimination.[39] Our BIPOC veterinary colleagues have made video reports, written articles, and shared their most painful and intimate stories of experiencing racism.[40] The least we can do is to listen to their stories and believe them. We owe our colleagues so much better than disbelief, color-blind ideology, or sympathy with no action for change. Our fellow veterinarians cannot change the color of their skin. We can change our understanding of ourselves, our understanding of racism, and our ability to work for justice.

ARE WE GOING TO TALK ABOUT WHITE PRIVILEGE?

It has always been possible to be a white veterinarian in the US and Canada. There has never been a time where a small white child could not find role models in veterinary medicine.[41] This is because we live in a country that was founded by and designed for the well-being, welfare, and success of white people like us. "White privilege" is just another way of saying "the people who look like you invented the thing, made the rules about the thing, and are winning at the thing they created."[42]

Another way to think about privilege is that it is a part of your identity that gives you access (or lack of barriers) to power and resources. For example, when you are white, that part of your identity accords you privilege because racism is not an additional obstacle placed in your path on the road to your future. Race is not the only part of your identity that can confer privilege. Gender, disability, veterinary experience, and student debt can make access to power and resources more or less challenging.

Social workers have used the idea of positioning oneself within a web of identities in order to understand yourself and how your identities intersect with one another (**Fig. 2**).[43] Use the web in **Fig. 2** to map out your own identities. In what aspects of your identity are you closest to power and resources? In what aspects of your identity do you experience barriers to accessing power and resources? How do the different parts of your identity intersect to shape your experience? While the focus of this article is largely on race and whiteness, your racial identity is inextricably intertwined with every other identity you have. How do your other identities affect how public policy (such as laws around family leave or access to mental health care) impacts you?

In order to create a veterinary profession where everyone can thrive and succeed, white veterinarians must look at our history and ourselves. If we can understand our own racial identity, we can better understand how race and racism operate and we can become more successful in shaping the future of the veterinary profession.

ARE YOU SURE BEING WHITE DOES NOT MAKE ME A BAD PERSON?

Here is one way to answer that question. My white ancestors did some horrific things. In the US and Canada, millions of Black Africans were enslaved and treated as property and millions of Native Americans were dispossessed of their land and killed.[16,44] It hurts to think about the idea that people I am related to and people who came before me doing truly unspeakable things, and that the legacy of the racist ideas that enabled

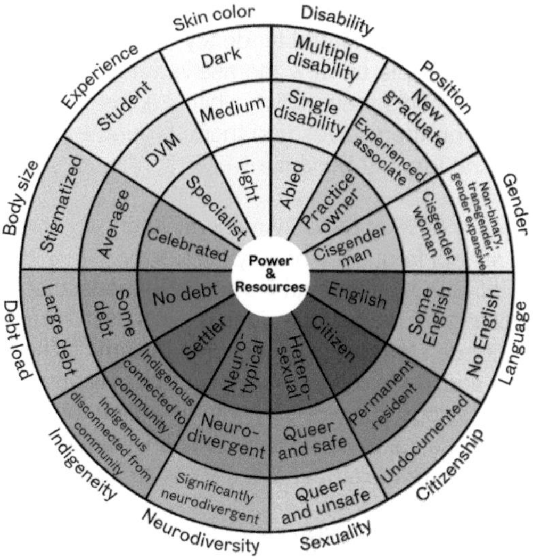

Fig. 2. Power Web. A power web is a way of mapping out your individual identities and thinking through where your identities are closer to power and resources. Each wedge of the web is a different facet of your identity. The closer to the center of the web, the fewer barriers between you and power or resources. You are a unique composition of identities. Not every part of your identity has equal weight; you might find that while several of your identities present more barriers between you and power or resources, your skin color (and race) act as a factor that remove many barriers. The shape of your web may change with time as your identities grow and evolve.

these choices persists today.[17] This does not make me a bad person for being white. I am not guilty of the things my ancestors did. I am the person who neither devised nor implemented segregation that prevented Black people from attending veterinary school. I am responsible for correcting the wrongs of the past, and I am responsible for living my life in a way that does not replicate those harmful patterns.[45]

The way we help right past wrongs is not by pretending we are not white or that race does not apply to us. It is by understanding what race is and is not, how it functions, and how we can be empowered by our own racial identity so that we can shape a better and brighter future and fulfill our sworn veterinary oath. By seeing ourselves and our whiteness, we can also see the people around us. In becoming grounded in our white identity, we can more clearly identify racist ideas, reject them, and counter them.

CLINICS CARE POINTS

- After reading this article, read each article in this issue.
- The challenges faced in our profession are not insurmountable, but they do require following the leadership of those most impacted by the problems of racism and discrimination.
- A diverse pantheon of leaders will lead to more novel, creative, and successful solutions.
- When a BIPOC author proposes a solution to the problems of discrimination, racism, and bigotry, believe them and implement the solution.

DISCLOSURE

The author has nothing to disclose.

REFERENCES

1. Bennett A. 'I don't have to Be perfect to do good. The Tyee; 2023. Available at: https://thetyee.ca/Culture/2023/10/06/Jess-Housty-Crushed-Wild-Mint-Heiltsuk-Coastal-Poetry/. [Accessed 9 February 2024].
2. Mills R. Perfection or Excellence: Which Is Your Quest? EyeNet Mag 2007;07:5.
3. Greenhill LM, Brandt J. 77: getting past the fear of talking about race. Available at: https://soundcloud.com/diversitymatters-at-aavmc/77-getting-past-the-fear-of-talking-about-race. [Accessed 18 February 2024].
4. Mukhopadhyay CC, Henze R, Moses YT. How real is race?: a sourcebook on race, culture, and biology. Lanham, MD: Rowman & Littlefield; 2013.
5. Kissinger K, Bohnhoff C. All the colors we are: the story of how we get our skin color = todos los colores de nuestra piel: La Historia de Por Qué Tenemos Diferentes Colores de Piel. 20th anniversary edition 2014. St. Paul, MN: Redleaf Press; 2014.
6. McChesney KY. Teaching Diversity: The Science You Need to Know to Explain Why Race Is Not Biological. Sage Open 2015;5(4). 2158244015611712.
7. Bhopal R. The beautiful skull and Blumenbach's errors: the birth of the scientific concept of race. BMJ 2007;335(7633):1308–9.
8. Fuentes A, Ackermann RR, Athreya S, et al. AAPA statement on race and racism. Am J Phys Anthropol 2019;169(3):400–2.
9. Cerdeña JP, Plaisime MV, Tsai J. From race-based to race-conscious medicine: how anti-racist uprisings call us to act. Lancet 2020;396(10257):1125–8.
10. Skinner-Dorkenoo AL, Rogbeer KG, Sarmal A, et al. Challenging Race-Based Medicine Through Historical Education About the Social Construction of Race. Health Equity 2023;7(1):764–72.
11. Khan AT, Gogarten SM, McHugh CP, et al. Recommendations on the use and reporting of race, ethnicity, and ancestry in genetic research: Experiences from the NHLBI TOPMed program. Cell Genomics 2022;2(8):100155.
12. Norton HL, Quillen EE, Bigham AW, et al. Human races are not like dog breeds: refuting a racist analogy. Evol Educ Outreach 2019;12(1):17.
13. Parker HG, Kim LV, Sutter NB, et al. Genetic structure of the purebred domestic dog. Science 2004;304(5674):1160–4.
14. McGhee HC. The sum of us: what racism costs everyone and how we can prosper together. 1st edition. New York, NY: One World; 2021.
15. Greenhill LM. Colorblindness is not a cure. Todays Vet Bus 2020;4(6):80–3.
16. Kendi IX. How to be an antiracist. One World; 2019.
17. Wilkerson I. Caste: the origins of our discontents. First edition. New York, NY: Random House; 2020.
18. Annual Data Report 2022-2023 American Association of Veterinary Medical Colleges. Washington, DC, Published online 2023.
19. JAVMA News. J Am Vet Med Assoc 2020;257(2):115–42.
20. JAVMA News. J Am Vet Med Assoc 2021;258(12):1289–316.
21. Labor Force Characteristics by Race and Ethnicity, 2014. Published online 2015.
22. Employment status of the Hispanic or Latino population by age and sex. Published online 2023.

23. Munroe M. The Need for Race Based Data in Canada. Univ Tor Med J 2022;99(3). Available at: https://jps.library.utoronto.ca/index.php/utmj/article/view/38223. [Accessed 16 February 2024].
24. Jones BV. The history of veterinary medicine and the animal-human relationship. Toronto, Ontario: 5m Books; 2021.
25. JAVMA News. J Am Vet Med Assoc 2011;238(1):8–26.
26. Miller EB. Private veterinary colleges in the United States, 1852-1927. J Am Vet Med Assoc 1981;178(6):583–93.
27. AVMA celebrates Black History Month by highlighting Black pioneers in veterinary medicine | American Veterinary Medical Association. 2021. Available at: https://www.avma.org/news/press-releases/avma-celebrates-black-history-month-highlighting-black-pioneers-veterinary. [Accessed 16 February 2024].
28. Adams EW. A historical overview of African American veterinarians in the United States, 1889- 2000. J Vet Med Educ 2004;31(4):409–13.
29. History of the AVMA. American Veterinary Medical Association. Available at: https://www.avma.org/about/history-avma. [Accessed 16 February 2024].
30. Greenhill L, Elmore R, Stewart S, et al. Fifty years in the life of veterinary students. J Vet Med Educ 2015;42(5):480–8.
31. Gill G, Singh B. Where do deans of veterinary medicine in the United States and Canada come from? Can Vet J Rev Veterinaire Can 2020;61(11):1187–96.
32. Smith DF. Veterinary legacy: a tribute to african-american deans in veterinary medicine. veterinary legacy. 2012. Available at: https://veterinarylegacy.blogspot.com/2012/02/tribute-to-african-american-deans-in.html. [Accessed 16 February 2024].
33. AVMA News. J Am Vet Med Assoc 2023;261(9):1281–95.
34. McPherson T. CVMA: 70 and going strong. Can Vet J 2018;59(3):221–2.
35. Elmore RG. Reasons for the lack of racial diversity in veterinary medicine. J Vet Med Educ 2004;31(4):414–6.
36. News and Views; Veterinary Medicine. The most racially segregated field in graduate education today. J Blacks High Educ 2003;42:18.
37. Ricketts R. Do better: spiritual activism for fighting and healing from white supremacy. New York, NY: First Atria Books Hardcover Edition. Atria Books; 2021.
38. Greenhill LM, Carmichael KP. Survey of college climates at all 28 US colleges and schools of veterinary medicine: preliminary findings. J Vet Med Educ 2014;41(2): 111–21.
39. Shastri T. Equity, diversity and inclusion survey results. Focus Ont Vet Med Assoc Mag 2023;42(1):18–22.
40. Burkhard MJ, Dawkins S, Knoblaugh SE, et al. Supporting diversity, equity, inclusion, and belonging to strengthen and position the veterinary profession for service, sustainability, excellence, and impact. J Am Vet Med Assoc 2022;260(11): 1283–90.
41. Amass SF. Representations of the veterinary profession in nonfiction children's books. J Am Vet Med Assoc 2011;238(9):1126–31.
42. McIntosh P. White privilege: unpacking the invisible knapsack (1989) 1. 1st edition. Routledge: On Privilege, Fraudulence, and Teaching As Learning; 2019. p. 29–34.
43. Sisneros J, Stakeman C, Joyner MC, et al, D of the D of SWCL. Critical multicultural social work. New York, NY: Oxford University Press; 2008.
44. Maynard R, Simpson LB. Rehearsals for living. Alfred A. Toronto, Ontario: Knopf Canada; 2022.
45. Krawec P, Estes N. Becoming kin: an indigenous call to unforgetting the past and reimagining our future. Minneapolis, MN: Broadleaf Books; 2022.

The Owner Will See You Now

The Road to Entrepreneurship for Diverse Veterinarians

George Robinson, DVM, MSPH

KEYWORDS

• Diversity • Entrepreneurship • Pivot • Resilience • Support

KEY POINTS

- Minority veterinarians compose only a small fraction of practice owners.
- Diverse veterinarians must overcome adversity to achieve their ownership goals.
- People, patience, processes, and pivoting provide a framework for practice ownership.
- Support and community are paramount to a diverse veterinary entrepreneur's success.
- Learning from your mistakes makes you a better veterinary practice owner.

INTRODUCTION

Veterinary medicine is one of the least racially diverse professions in America. Estimates from The Bureau of Labor Statistics indicate that 90% of veterinarians identify as white, a statistical that only recently has been recognized as a problem.[1] Many diverse veterinarians who enter the profession face different challenges than those from mostly white backgrounds, which can influence their career trajectory and discourage them from becoming practice or business owners. Although no statistics are available about the number of veterinary practices owned by racial minorities, we can surmise from general business statistics that the number is likely low. According to 2022 US Census data, 21% of businesses are minority-owned, with "minority" defined as any race or ethnicity combination not classified as white or non-Hispanic.[2]

We know that increasing diversity has positive effects, but we also know that we must expose under-represented students to the veterinary profession at a young age. Currently, diversity, equity, and inclusion interventions are focused on creating and supporting more diverse veterinarians who can serve as role models for future generations. I argue that we must go further by encouraging and supporting minorities on their path to veterinary entrepreneurship.

Founder and Former CEO, Heartland Veterinary Partners, LLC, 10278 Porto Romano Drive, Miromar Lakes, FL 33913, USA
E-mail address: drgeorge.robinson@gmail.com

Vet Clin Small Anim 54 (2024) 849–858
https://doi.org/10.1016/j.cvsm.2024.06.008 **vetsmall.theclinics.com**
0195-5616/24/

Diversity starts at the top. When veterinary leadership and practice owner diversity increase, we're likely to see a trickle-down effect that will attract more non-white veterinarians to a profession that understands and acknowledges their unique needs, the challenges they faced to get where they are, and the continual challenges surrounding race that lie ahead.

As a successful African American veterinary entrepreneur, I have faced my fair share of adversity. The road to success was not always smooth, but I stayed laser-focused on my long-term goals and simultaneously learned how to pivot and embrace setbacks. Although my inherent persistence certainly played a role, I would not be where I am today without the help of other minority veterinarians and business owners who paved the way and welcomed me into the fold.

MY STORY

I grew up in a family of intellectuals, academics, and business owners. My father was the Chairman of the Animal Science Department and interim Dean of the College of Agriculture at Southern University in Baton Rouge, LA, and I was raised in an environment that nurtured my natural intelligence and curiosity. When I decided as a teenager I wanted to become a veterinarian, I didn't see any reason why I couldn't.

So, I went to vet school. In 1981, I was the first African American Louisiana resident to graduate from Louisiana State University's School of Veterinary Medicine. After veterinary school, I considered a public health career, among other job options, so I completed a master's degree in public health at Howard University. My thoughts were that I would pursue all of my educational options before starting my career. Afterward, however, I struggled to find a public health job or a position in industry and decided to enter general veterinary practice instead. When I lost my first job after about a year, I wasn't sure what to do. Then, a client called and asked if I could care for her pet, and I realized that if New Orleans had only limited opportunities for me, I should create my own.

I opened a house-call practice and became the first African American veterinary practice owner in New Orleans. I eventually moved to a brick-and-mortar location where I practiced for many years and was heavily involved in the community—but, as one does, I eventually burned out. I decided I no longer wanted to deal with the pressures of practice ownership, sold the practice, and moved to Atlanta to practice as an associate. Eventually, my skills as a manager and leader were recognized and I lived in Florida, California, and Chicago managing several large, multi-unit group practices.

As those practices grew, I slowly became disillusioned with the direction I saw that private equity firms were leading veterinarians. I could see no path to retribution for the company I worked for at the time, so I decided to leave. I felt that a veterinarian-led company would perform better. I started Heartland Veterinary Partners to try to fix problems I saw with corporate veterinary medicine.

Heartland grew rapidly because of our vet-centric, hands-off model, and we sold to a larger private equity group in 2019 to increase our resources and continue to grow. I stepped down as chief executive officer but remained on Heartland's board of directors to advise the company, particularly for growth and development of the company culture. I am also passionate about supporting and mentoring other African American students and veterinarians in my spare time.

LIGHTING THE SPARK

I was always business-minded, and I wanted to become an entrepreneur from a young age. I also knew I wanted to become a veterinarian, but simply earning a Doctor of

Veterinary Medicine (DVM) degree was not good enough—I wanted to become the wealthiest African American veterinarian. I may have been onto something because, according to a 2016 study, the wealth gap between white Americans and minorities is projected to only increase. The study found that the average annual wealth increase for white Americans in the 30 years prior was $18,000, compared with only $750 for black Americans.[3]

I didn't buy into the narrative of the starving, selfless veterinarian charging pennies (or not charging) because "It's not about the money." My veterinary school professors tried to lower my expectations, but they weren't entrepreneurs and I made a point of not internalizing their lack of encouragement. Being successful, financially comfortable, and a compassionate veterinarian making a difference in the world are not mutually exclusive.

I began consuming any business information I could get and learned about Dr Matthew Jenkins, a Tuskegee Veterinary School graduate operating a lucrative California practice. I wanted to go straight to the source, so I wrote to him, and in a serendipitous turn of events, he wrote back with an invitation to California. I obliged. Dr Jenkins had already sold his successful practice, and I wanted to do the same as he did, but better. I did a preceptorship under the new ownership at his former practice and was mentored by the 2 outstanding African American veterinarians who helped build my business and medical knowledge.

That infusion of grassroots knowledge helped to motivate me and to recognize and address my weaknesses, so I could be a successful businessman going forward. Dr Jenkins and his practice set the bar, but other people guided, supported, and encouraged me along the way. To pay it forward, I started a scholarship at LSU to create a new generation of African American veterinarians, and I travel to veterinary schools and conferences to motivate and inspire those on their career journeys.

OVERCOMING ROADBLOCKS FOR DIVERSE VETERINARIANS

Becoming an entrepreneur is a challenging feat for anyone, but minorities face a unique set of roadblocks to achieve their goals. Here, I explore common scenarios a diverse veterinarian may encounter on their journey and ways to go over, around, or through them.

The Impact of Discrimination

When I started out, finding a job was difficult, and I felt that racial discrimination was the reason. But, I did not act like a victim or emotionally shut down. Instead, I took the opportunity to do something positive. It was what it was, so I opened my first practice when the opportunity arose. In today's society, you shouldn't have to worry about discrimination, but the unfortunate reality is that you will face it in some way, shape, or form during your career. An Intuit Quickbooks study found that 79% of black business owners have experienced racism from a customer, and 82% have changed their behavior around customers and vendors to avoid negative stereotypes.[4]

The Power of Demographics

A demographic study is part of every good business plan and can help you deal with potential discrimination or biases among pet owners and other community veterinary professionals. As a minority, you will attract clients specifically because of your race or ethnicity. You'll also see a subset of people who assume the quality of your services is lower, or the competition will cast you in an unfavorable light. Racism is everywhere, but choosing your location wisely can minimize negative effects. Alternatively, choosing the wrong location can be disastrous.

Consumer intelligence technology is essential in solidifying your business plan. By analyzing local income levels via a demographic study, you can quantify your business plan and predict your intended or desired practice style. If the average area income is low, consider crafting a low-cost, high-volume model that meets the community's needs. If income levels are higher, you can support a high-quality, low-volume model and expect a high average client transaction. However, you must also consider whether that area's residents may not use your services because of your race. Then, you may bring in less income than anticipated and find yourself in a precarious financial position.

Obtaining Business Capital

Securing capital is another pivotal step for a diverse veterinarian on the path to entrepreneurship. I had great difficulty obtaining capital, because the banks simply didn't lend to minorities. While this has improved because many major banking institutions now have diversity initiatives, a 2023 Intuit Quickbooks survey found that 57% of black business owners were denied business loans at least once, compared with 37% of non-black applicants. The survey also found that once approved for a loan, black business owners spent $5000 more to start their businesses compared with non-black start-ups.[4]

An outstanding business plan is paramount to improve your chances of loan approval. Biases against minorities—whether conscious or unconscious—impact lending decisions, and you must go above and beyond to prove that your business is a good investment. A solid business plan not only helps you secure capital, but also serves as a blueprint for business development and growth.

You don't need an MBA to learn what creating a new business involves or how to write a stand-out business plan that provides realistic projections of expected income and expenses for the first 3 to 5 years. Plenty of quality resources are available for free or purchase on the internet, including books, websites, and online courses, which leaves no room for excuses for failing to educate yourself. In a Bank of America Survey, 56% of black business owners said they were self-taught.[5] Start on the right foot by ensuring you thoroughly understand what's to come.

While creating a business plan and applying for loans, entrepreneurs commonly make the mistake of estimating or accepting too little capital to support them during the early years. You must project your expected income and losses realistically and accurately to ensure you have enough to get through the first few business years comfortably. Comfortably—not scraping by.

Veterinary practices require astronomical overhead that requires loans that can look insurmountable. But, if you've committed to practice ownership, done your due diligence, and developed a viable business plan, you must trust that you'll eventually see a return on your investment. Never underestimate your capital needs, because losing money while you try to grow your new business has significant negative impacts. Your stress level will rise and spill over to your employees, and your personal life may suffer. Of course, once secured, you must use the capital wisely.

Alleviating Student Debt Fears

Because practice ownership loans are so large, many fresh veterinary graduates—who likely already carry large student debt—shy away from the idea of practice ownership, or entrepreneurship in general. This is especially true of minority veterinarians, who statistically more likely will have fewer available resources or grew up in poverty because of long-standing systemic racial inequalities.[6]

Don't let your student debt scare you. If you plan to wait to start or purchase a business until you have paid off a significant portion of your debt, you may never get there. In the long term, a practice owner's earnings potential is equal to or greater than a non-owner associate, although you may have to weather a few years of lower pay before reaching your full potential. According to American Veterinary Medical Association (AVMA) data, the average associate salary in 2022 was $141,000, compared with the average practice owner's salary of $191,000.[7] Your student debt does not have to stand in the way of entrepreneurship.

Finding Social Support

Trying to run a minority-owned business without a strong support system can feel lonely and isolating. You can connect with majority business owners, but they won't always understand how your diverse status impacts business operations and how customers treat you. Or, you can connect with other minority friends or family members, but they are unlikely to understand the business side of your struggles. Still, fight the urge to go it alone and instead make finding a trusted community of experienced minority and majority business owners a priority. Whether or not that community is in the veterinary space, being able to turn to the group with questions or ideas is invaluable. Be selective in choosing your group, ensuring they offer a supportive environment that will help you thrive, and that they can provide factual information and insights into running a business.

THE FOUR "Ps" FOR MINORITY ENTREPRENEURS

One of my favorite concepts that I emphasize when I discuss business strategy is the 3 P's, or in this case, 4—people, process, patience, and pivot. The P's can apply to nearly any business situation and clever alliteration makes them memorable. As with most other business efforts, diverse entrepreneurs can benefit from applying these strategies, but they must apply them well, since they are often judged more harshly than their majority counterparts.

I learned the 3 P's the hard way, as most business owners do. I tried things the way I thought was best, failed, and regrouped to try again. Every failure should be considered a positive, and provided that you learn from it, you can move forward with more knowledge and a better plan.

People

People are the single most important asset of any business enterprise—especially a veterinary practice. You can purchase only the most expensive equipment and build a multi-million dollar facility, but your business will be only as good as the people working inside. Choosing the right team members, paying them adequately, coaching and developing them to grow with the business are important steps on your journey. Treat your team members well, and they'll reward you with loyalty and hard work.

You must invest in your people to grow and sustain a business and, if you haven't already noticed—veterinary medicine is a relatively small field. According to 2023 AVMA data, the profession currently supports only 127,131 veterinarians.[8] So, making lasting connections with other veterinary professionals is important for building a support system and network of colleagues who can help you when you need it.

Processes

Keep the next P—processes—in mind as you pursue your entrepreneurial goals. Once you have the right people in place, you need to create processes and protocols to help the business run, and you and your team must execute them well. Processes should be individualized to your practice style and long-term goals, should help create consistency for employees and clients, and should ensure important steps don't fall through the cracks. The more processes you can standardize—from medical protocols to management and accounting—the smoother your business will run and the easier new team members can be onboarded.

Personal processes are also important to your success as a minority entrepreneur. You'll find that most of the time you're juggling a million tasks and struggling to keep them in check. Hiring a practice manager is best, but may not be possible early in your business endeavors, so you must find a way to stay organized.

I found the Eisenhower matrix a helpful tool for prioritizing tasks. The technique, which uses 4 boxes to categorize tasks according to their urgency and importance, was introduced to me by an attorney friend who sensed that I was struggling early in my career. I lived the concept, found it helpful, and successfully incorporated it into my daily scheduling and career planning. A plethora of scheduling and productivity tools are available in mobile app and desktop formats, some of which use the Eisenhower matrix or other popular techniques. I recommend trying several and finding which works best for your unique brain.

Establishing routines at work and home can help prevent burnout. Most new or aspiring business owners do too much for too long, which can lead to a poor work-life balance and problems at home. Set specific work hours and stick to them to ensure you can recharge before returning to work. Do not forget to incorporate movement into your days or weeks—something you truly enjoy and that makes you feel great—to reduce stress.

Patience

I've worked in or managed many veterinary practices in nearly every US state and I've seen first-hand some of the biggest problems plaguing their teams. I often see interpersonal conflict because of a lack of patience, which has also been a personal struggle. Veterinarians are smart and busy people, who can easily become frustrated and impatient with untrained staff members who are causing them stress, and then they act out negatively toward an employee simply trying to do their job. When tension develops between veterinarians and their team members, you will see high turnover rates and an incohesive team culture.

Early in my career, I failed to recognize that my people, and my investment of time and energy in their development, were so important. I knew my staff weren't happy, but I didn't realize how unhappy. One Christmas morning, I found myself working entirely alone, because my staff had walked out. I never took my anxieties or frustrations out on the staff again.

I also want to mention the importance of being patient with yourself and your business. Whatever your vision, remember it will take time to execute—especially if you want to do it well. Give yourself grace and set realistic goals and expectations. Be kind to yourself, because not everyone else will.

Resiliency and the Pivot

The final P is a big one—Pivot. This concept has followed me through my long and winding career, reminding me to embrace change instead of fighting it. Throughout your veterinary career, you will be faced with many decision points at which you can pivot and adapt, or continue to struggle. Recognizing when to push on and when to cut your losses comes with experience and requires that you remain true and kind to yourself.

There will be times in your practice, team, personal, or entrepreneurial development when you are forced to pivot for any number of reasons. Although change is never easy, I recognize that my career has been so varied because I didn't fear the pivot. I said "Yes" to advancement opportunities, despite the fact that some required cross-country moves, and I created my own opportunities when I felt I needed change in my life.

At times, I've embraced the pivot to correct a misstep. The day my entire staff quit, I knew I had to make a major change in how I presented myself, how I ran my practice, and how I treated people. Sometimes you need a slap in the face to see what has been there all along, and as much as it felt bad at the time, it made me become a better practice owner, manager, mentor, and friend.

It was clear that I had to pivot. The proof was in the pudding—the way I managed my team and hospital wasn't working. I had to look in the mirror and assess the situation. Was I the problem? What could I do to be a better leader, increase employee retention, and spark employee engagement? One of the few things you can change about your environment and circumstances is yourself.

I have been committed to the pivot since that event. Now, I do more listening than talking, I make an effort to cultivate empathy, and I think twice before raising my voice. I've seen the difference first-hand, and truly believe the power of the pivot made me a better leader and got me where I am today.

FINANCIAL ACCOUNTABILITY

Profitability is a dirty word in veterinary school. Students and professors avoid talking about the money aspect of practice, but in real life, profit is everything. Owning a business is a huge responsibility and your shoulders will carry considerable weight as you worry about making your employee payroll, with enough left to sustain yourself and your family.

You can allay some of the burden of managing business finances by ensuring you have a solid grasp of your current situation. When you know exactly where you stand, you can take control and right the ship if necessary, but not knowing only breeds more anxiety. At the end of the day, profit is the most important thing, but that isn't the same as revenue. Your total revenue goes to various routine operational expenses, but profit determines your company's worth, the amount you can invest in yourself or back into the business, and your business's overall health.

If you aren't making a profit, you must critically re-evaluate your operations. Ideally, you'll save yourself from this situation with a thorough business plan and a pro forma that accurately predicts your likely profit and loss. Then, you must take the area's demographics into account and use your financial projections to price your goods and services appropriately to keep you afloat in a comfortable place.

THE PRESSURE TO PERFORM

Good bookkeeping and accounting are essential to accurately determine your financial status, but equally important for diverse entrepreneurs is finding someone who will share their ups, downs, failures, and triumphs. As I previously mentioned, the veterinary space is small, and the minority veterinary space is even smaller. You may feel pressure from your colleagues or from inside yourself to do well and represent your community in a positive light. So, you grit your teeth and smile, and tell everyone that things have been great.

This pressure can add a layer of stress that, as a minority practice owner, you surely do not need. Finding a confidant, ideally another minority business owner, who can share your ups and downs will help you both stay sane and keep you accountable to your goals.

EXPERT TIPS TO HELP DIVERSE VETERINARIANS THRIVE

I know first-hand that breaking down barriers and forging a rarely traveled path can be extremely difficult. Here are a few things I've learned over the years that significantly impacted my success as an African American veterinary entrepreneur.

Become a Self-Guided Learner

When I was growing up, the internet was not readily available to point me toward the resources and information I needed to achieve my goal of entrepreneurship in veterinary medicine. Instead, I found others who had walked a similar path and I went straight to the source to learn. Take charge of your future by reading everything you can, watching webinars and videos, and speaking to experienced business owners.

Gather a Team

As much as some of us believe it's possible, nobody can or should run a business entirely on their own. You need a team, which should include your family and friends, your veterinary colleagues and employees, and your accountant, lawyer, and practice or business consultants, to support you on your road to entrepreneurship. Don't be afraid to reach out for help, because nobody except yourself expects you to know everything!

Surround Yourself with Community

Some people on your path will brush you off and underestimate you based on negative perceptions of your minority status, which can lead to feelings of exclusion. When you feel left out, isolation becomes the next logical step, but this is never the answer and typically makes things worse. When I first started in veterinary school, I was the only African American in my class. I tried hard to keep my head down, and always went straight home after class, but the result was that I struggled to compete with the other students, who spent time studying and collaborating to enhance their learning. When I integrated myself into the community, my grades and performance immediately improved.

If you are not surrounded by a diversity-minded business or veterinary community, consider joining or creating a virtual community. Social media makes it easy to connect with like-minded individuals, especially business-based platforms. However, keep an eye out for misinformation and distracting videos that could derail your intentions.

Learn to Embrace Failure

Growing up, I thought failure was not an option. I lived my life in this perfectionistic state for years, until I was forced to deal with my many failures as I grew my businesses. Over time, you learn that you cannot possibly be successful at everything and you must learn to manage, rather than avoid, failure. As long as you can step back and learn from your mistakes, trying something that doesn't work is OK. Don't let the fear of failure hold you back from becoming a veterinary entrepreneur.

Take Pride in Your Achievements

Racism and other biases aren't going away anytime soon. Some people hear or see certain adjectives before a doctor's name and automatically make negative assumptions about that person. I spent my early career trying not to draw attention to myself and my many accomplishments, until a client pointed out that if I wanted respect for what I'd achieved rather than disrespect because of my skin, I needed to show the world how great I was. Since then, I've made sure to introduce myself as "doctor" and I proudly display my degrees and accolades for all to see. You see, I am somewhat of a big deal, and so are you. Let the world know!

Every diverse veterinarian has overcome adversity to get where they are. You need to make known what you've accomplished despite that adversity, because nobody will do this but you.

SUMMARY

Given the small number of diverse veterinarians and separately diverse business owners, we can assume that only a few minority veterinarians make the leap into entrepreneurship. To expand diversity in the profession, we must not discourage minority vets from pursuing practice ownership and other business endeavors, and we must start supporting those who seek to break the mold. Because biases and racism still exist in business, prospective entrepreneurs must acknowledge the difficulties they face and seek help from like-minded individuals and communities to overcome common roadblocks on the path to veterinary practice ownership. Prospective entrepreneurs should also take pride in their achievements, make an effort to stand out from the crowd in a positive way, and employ tried-and-true business strategies to ensure success.

CLINICS CARE POINTS

- Minority veterinarians interested in entrepreneurship must commit to overcoming diversity-specific roadblocks.
- In the United States, 10% of veterinarians and 21% of business owners are classified as racial minorities. Assuming a similar distribution of veterinary practice owners, we can surmise that only 2% of veterinary practice owners are non-white.
- Diverse entrepreneurs can benefit from applying the 4 P's—people, processes, patience, and pivot—to business strategies.

DISCLOSURE

The author has nothing to disclose.

REFERENCES

1. Bureau of Labor Statistics. Labor Force Statistics from the Current Population Survey. U.S. Department of Labor. Available at: https://www.bls.gov/cps/cpsaat11.htm. [Accessed 27 March 2024].
2. United States Census Bureau. Annual business survey shows employer and business characteristics. U.S. Department of Commerce; 2023. Available at: https://www.census.gov/newsroom/press-releases/2023/annual-business-survey-employer-business-characteristics.html. [Accessed 27 March 2024].
3. Asante-Muhammad D, Collins C, Hoxie J, et al. The ever-growing gap: failing to address the status quo will make closing the racial wealth gap impossible. Washington, DC: Institute for Policy Studies; 2016. Available at: https://ips-dc.org/wp-content/uploads/2016/08/The-Ever-Growing-Gap-CFED_IPS-Final-2.pdf. [Accessed 27 March 2024].

4. QuickBooks. Black history month survey 2023: insights for small businesses. Mountain View (CA): Intuit Inc.; 2023. Available at: https://quickbooks.intuit.com/r/small-business-data/black-history-month-survey-2023/. [Accessed 27 March 2024].
5. Bank of America. Women + minority business owner spotlight. Bank of America Corporation; 2022. Available at: https://about.bankofamerica.com/en/making-an-impact/women-and-minority-business-spotlight-2023. [Accessed 27 March 2024].
6. United States Census Bureau. Poverty rates for blacks and hispanics reached historic lows in 2019. U.S. Department of Commerce; 2020. Available at: https://www.census.gov/library/stories/2020/09/poverty-rates-for-blacks-and-hispanics-reached-historic-lows-in-2019.html. [Accessed 27 March 2024].
7. American Veterinary Medical Association. Veterinarian Salaries Struggle to Keep Up with Inflation. Schaumburg, IL: American Veterinary Medical Association. Available at: https://www.avma.org/news/veterinarian-salaries-struggle-keep-inflation. [Accessed 27 March 2024].
8. American Veterinary Medical Association. Market Research Statistics: U.S. Veterinarians. American Veterinary Medical Association. Available at: https://www.avma.org/resources-tools/reports-statistics/market-research-statistics-us-veterinarians. [Accessed 27 March 2024].

SUGGESTED READING

Ackerman L, Tilley L. Blackwell's five-minute veterinary practice management consult. 2nd edition. Ames (IA): Wiley-Blackwell; 2013.

Donnelly AL. 101 veterinary practice management questions answered. Ames (IA): Wiley-Blackwell; 2010.

Donnelly AL. Leading and managing veterinary teams: the definitive guide to veterinary practice management. Ames (IA): Wiley-Blackwell; 2006.

Gerber ME. The E Myth revisited: why most small businesses don't work and what to do about it. New York: HarperBusiness; 1995.

Gerber ME, Weinstein P. The E-Myth veterinarian. New York: HarperCollins; 2015.

Heinke ML. Practice made perfect: a complete guide to veterinary practice management. Ames (IA): Wiley-Blackwell; 2013.

Multicultural Veterinary Medical Association. Available at: mcvma.org.

National Association of Black Veterinarians. Available at: nabvonline.org.

Newfield A. Oops, I became a manager: managing the veterinary hospital team by finding unicorns (the oops management series). Trenton (NJ): AAHA Press; 2020.

Seibert P, Catanzaro TE. Veterinary practice management secrets. Philadelphia: Hanley & Belfus; 2002.

9780443297182